Table of Contents

CME Information

Release/Expiration Dates
Released: July, 2016
CME credit expires: July, 2019

Overview
Sleep was once described as a vital behavior of unknown function. Although there is still much debate regarding the exact function of sleep, over the past decade, our understanding of the molecular and biological processes that underlie sleep and wake states has increased exponentially. Likewise, we have become ever more aware of the physiological and psychiatric consequences of disturbed sleep. In this book, we provide an update on the current knowledge of the environmental, neurobiological, and genetic factors that influence sleep and wakefulness. We also provide evidence-based guidance for the accurate diagnosis and optimal treatment of various sleep/wake disorders.

Learning Objectives
After completing this activity, you should be better able to:

- Describe the neurobiological and molecular bases of sleep/wake cycles
- Apply differential diagnostic assessment of patients with sleep/wake problems according to established best practices
- Implement treatment strategies to address sleep/wake disorders

Accreditation and Credit Designation Statements

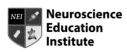 **Neuroscience Education Institute**

The Neuroscience Education Institute is accredited by the Accreditation Council for Continuing Medical Education (ACCME) to provide continuing medical education for physicians.

The Neuroscience Education Institute designates this enduring material for a maximum of 6.0 *AMA PRA Category 1 Credits*™. Physicians should claim only the credit commensurate with the extent of their participation in the activity.

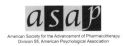

American Society for the Advancement of Pharmacotherapy
Division 55, American Psychological Association

The American Society for the Advancement of Pharmacotherapy (ASAP), Division 55 of the American Psychological Association, is approved by the American Psychological Association to sponsor continuing education for psychologists. ASAP maintains responsibility for this program and its content.

The American Society for the Advancement of Pharmacotherapy designates this program for 6.0 CE credits for psychologists.

Nurses: for all of your CNE requirements for recertification, the ANCC will accept *AMA PRA Category 1 Credits™* from organizations accredited by the ACCME. Some of the content of this activity pertains to pharmacology and is worth 2.0 continuing education hours of pharmacotherapeutics.

Physician Assistants: the NCCPA accepts *AMA PRA Category 1 Credits™* from organizations accredited by the AMA (providers accredited by the ACCME).

Optional Posttest and CME Credit Instructions
There is a fee for the optional posttest (waived for NEI Members). The estimated time for completion of this activity is 6.0 hours.

1. <u>Read the book</u>, evaluating the content presented
2. <u>Complete the posttest</u> and evaluation, available only online at **www.neiglobal.com/CME** (under "Book")
3. <u>Print your certificate</u> (if a score of 70% or more is achieved)

Questions? call 888-535-5600, or email CustomerService@neiglobal.com

Peer Review
This material has been peer-reviewed by a clinician specializing in sleep disorders to ensure the scientific accuracy and medical relevance of information presented and its independence from commercial bias. The Neuroscience Education Institute takes responsibility for the content, quality, and scientific integrity of this CME activity.

Disclosures

It is the policy of NEI to ensure balance, independence, objectivity, and scientific rigor in all its educational activities. Therefore, all individuals in a position to influence or control content are required to disclose any financial relationships. Although potential conflicts of interest are identified and resolved prior to the activity being presented, it remains for the participant to determine whether outside interests reflect a possible bias in either the exposition or the conclusions presented.

Disclosed financial relationships with conflicts of interest have been reviewed by the NEI CME Advisory Board Chair and resolved.

Author/Developer
Debbi Ann Morrissette, PhD
Adjunct Professor, Biological Sciences, Palomar College, San Marcos, CA
Senior Medical Writer, Neuroscience Education Institute, Carlsbad, CA
No financial relationships to disclose.

Content Editor
Stephen M. Stahl, MD, PhD
Adjunct Professor, Department of Psychiatry, University of California, San Diego School of Medicine, La Jolla, CA
Honorary Visiting Senior Fellow, University of Cambridge, Cambridge, UK
Director of Psychopharmacology, California Department of State Hospitals, Sacramento, CA
Grant/Research: Acadia, Actavis/Allergan, Alkermes, Arbor, Avanir, Axovant, Biogen, Celgene, Forest, Forum, Jazz, Lilly, Lundbeck, Merck, Otsuka, Reviva, Servier, Shire, Sprout, Sunovion, Takeda, Teva, Tonix, Vanda
Consultant/Advisor: Acadia, Alkermes, Allergan, Arbor, Avanir, Axovant, Axsome, Biogen, Celgene, Forest, Forum/EnVivo, Genomind, Jazz, Lundbeck, Merck, Otsuka, Pamlab, Pierre Fabre, Reviva, Servier, Shire, Sprout, Sunovion, Takeda, Teva, Tonix, Vanda
Speakers Bureau: Forum, Lundbeck, Otsuka, Servier, Sunovion, Takeda
Board Member: Genomind

Peer Reviewer
Thomas Roth, PhD
Director, Sleep Disorders and Research Center, Henry Ford Hospital, Detroit, MI
Consultant/Advisor: Cerêve, Eisai, Flamel, Ipsen, Jazz, MEDACorp / Leerink Swann, Merck, NovaDel, Novartis, Pernix, Pfizer, Respironics, SEQ, Takeda
Speakers Bureau: Merck, Pernix

The **Design Staff** has no financial relationships to disclose.

Disclosure of Off-Label Use
This educational activity may include discussion of unlabeled and/or investigational uses of agents that are not currently labeled for such use by the FDA. Please consult the product prescribing information for full disclosure of labeled uses.

Disclaimer
Participants have an implied responsibility to use the newly acquired information from this activity to enhance patient outcomes and their own professional development. The information presented in this educational activity is not meant to serve as a guideline for patient management. Any procedures, medications, or other courses of diagnosis or treatment discussed or suggested in this educational activity should not be used by clinicians without evaluation of their patients' conditions and possible contraindications or dangers in use, review of any applicable manufacturer's product information, and comparison with recommendations of other authorities. Primary references and full prescribing information should be consulted.

Cultural and Linguistic Competency:
A variety of resources addressing cultural and linguistic competency can be found at this link: nei.global/CMEregs

Provider
This activity is provided by the Neuroscience Education Institute.
Additionally provided by the American Society for the Advancement of Pharmacotherapy.

Support
This activity is supported solely by the provider, Neuroscience Education Institute.

Stahl's Illustrated | Objectives

- Identify the neurobiological and molecular bases of sleep/wake cycles

- Apply differential diagnostic assessment of patients with sleep/wake problems according to established best practices

- Implement treatment strategies to address sleep/wake disorders

Stahl's Illustrated

Introduction

Sleep was once described as a vital behavior of unknown function (Roth and Roehrs, 2000). Although there is still much debate regarding the exact function of sleep, over the past decade, our understanding of the molecular and biological processes that underlie sleep and wake states have increased exponentially. Likewise, we have become ever more aware of the physiological and psychiatric consequences of disturbed sleep. In this book, we provide an update on the current knowledge of the environmental, neurobiological, and genetic factors that influence sleep and wakefulness. We also provide evidence-based guidance for the accurate diagnosis and optimal treatment of various sleep/wake disorders.

Neurobiology and Genetics of Sleep/Wake Disorders

In Chapter 1, we address the sleep/wake cycle and how this circadian behavior is affected by a myriad of neurotransmitter systems. We also discuss the molecular clock, a series of interacting transcription factors that influence sleep and many other physiological processes, and how genetic variation in molecular clock components may influence the sleep/wake cycle as well as cardiometabolic health, mental illness propensity, and risk of cancer. We hope that this chapter will convey the importance of sleep to whole body wellness so that readers will more enthusiastically appreciate the need for accurate diagnosis (Chapter 2) and appropriate treatment (Chapter 3) when the sleep/wake cycle is disrupted.

Epidemiology and Costs of Sleep/Wake Disorders

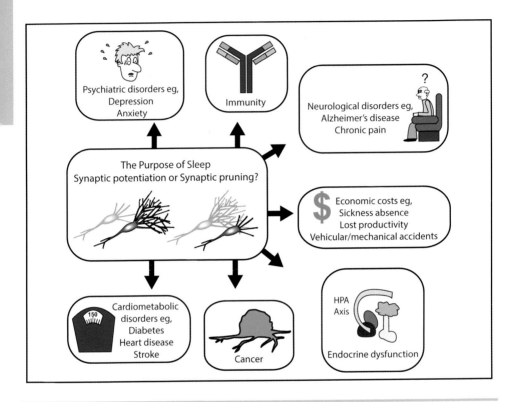

FIGURE 1.1. There is still much debate over the purpose of sleep. Some propose that sleep is essential for synaptic growth, while others argue that sleep is necessary for synaptic pruning (Mignot, 2012; Dresler et al., 2014). Regardless of which hypothesis—or some combination of both—is more accurate, it has become increasingly evident that disturbances of the sleep/wake cycle have a detrimental effect on a myriad of physiological and psychiatric functions. Aside from the economic costs of sleep/wake disorders, the risk of cardiometabolic disease, cancer, mental illness, and overall poorer quality of life are all increased when the sleep/wake cycle is disturbed (Cappuccio et al., 2010; Guo et al., 2013; Lallukka et al., 2014; Liu et al., 2013; Ohayon, 2012; Palma et al., 2013; Pigeon et al., 2012).

Sleep: How Much Is Too Much?
Too Little?

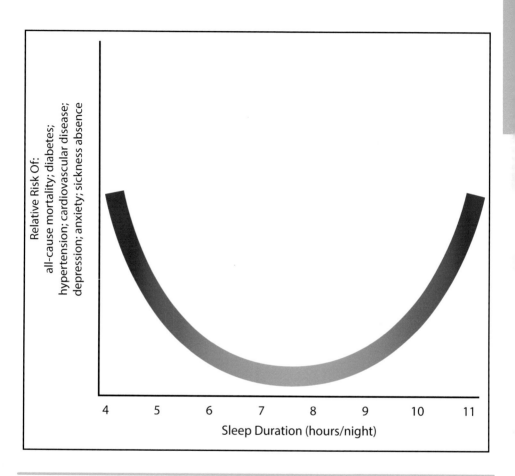

FIGURE 1.2. Both a short duration (<7 hours/night) and a long duration (>9 hours/night) of sleep have been associated with a variety of physiological and psychiatric illnesses, such as diabetes and depression, as well as an increased risk of death (Cappuccio et al., 2010; Guo et al., 2013; Lallukka et al., 2014; Liu et al., 2013). These data, represented here as a U-shaped curve, depict the sleep/wake cycle as a homeostatic process that requires a careful balance in order to maintain optimal health.

Arousal Spectrum

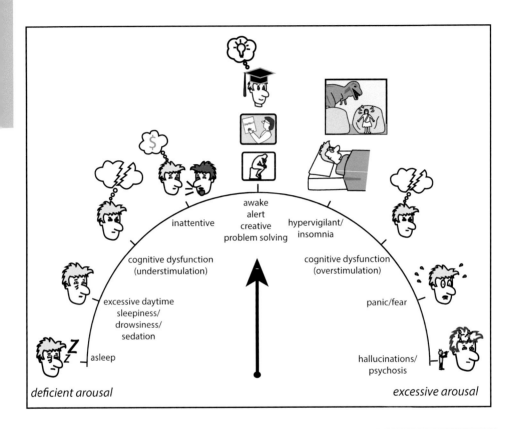

FIGURE 1.3. One's state of arousal is more complicated than simply being awake or asleep. Arousal exists as if on a dimmer switch, with many phases along the spectrum. Where on the spectrum one lies is largely influenced by 5 key neurotransmitters: histamine, dopamine, norepinephrine, serotonin, and acetylcholine. When there is balance between too much and too little arousal, one is awake, alert, and able to function well. As the dial shifts to the right, there is too much arousal, which may cause hypervigilance and consequently insomnia at night. Further increases in arousal can cause cognitive dysfunction, panic, and in extreme cases hallucinations. On the other hand, as arousal diminishes, individuals may experience inattentiveness, cognitive dysfunction, sleepiness, and ultimately sleep (Stahl, 2013).

The Sleep/Wake Cycle

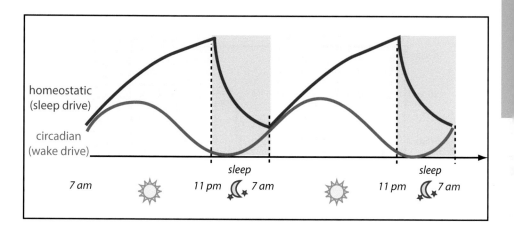

FIGURE 1.4. The sleep/wake cycle is mediated by 2 opposing drives: the homeostatic sleep drive and the circadian wake drive. The homeostatic drive accumulates throughout periods of wakefulness and is opposed by the circadian drive. The longer an individual is awake, the greater the homeostatic drive (Krystal et al., 2010). The homeostatic drive is dependent upon the accumulation of adenosine, which leads to the disinhibition of the ventrolateral preoptic (VLPO) nucleus and the release of GABA/galanin as part of the sleep circuit. The circadian drive, mediated by light acting upon the suprachiasmatic nucleus (SCN), stimulates the release of hypocretin/orexin as part of the wake circuit (Wulff et al., 2010).

The Sleep Cycle

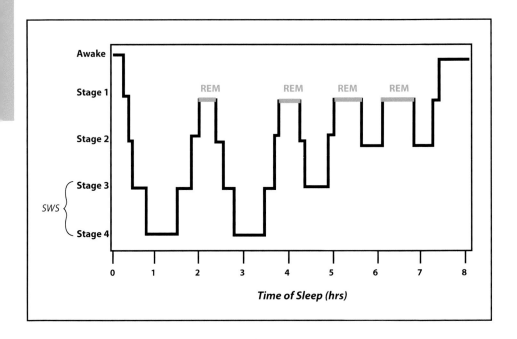

FIGURE 1.5. The complete sleep cycle (non-REM and REM) lasts approximately 90 minutes and occurs 4 to 5 times a night (Reeve and Bailes, 2010). Stages 1 and 2 comprise non-REM sleep, whereas stages 3 and 4 are part of deeper, slow-wave sleep (SWS) (Tafti, 2009). During the normal sleep period, the duration of non-REM sleep is gradually reduced while the duration of REM sleep is increased. REM sleep is characterized by faster activity on an electroencephalogram (EEG)—similar to that seen during periods of wakefulness—as well as distinct eye movements and peripheral muscle atonia. It is during REM sleep that dreaming occurs, and PET studies have shown activation of the thalamus, the visual cortex, and limbic regions accompanied by reduced metabolism in other regions, such as the dorsolateral prefrontal cortex (DLPFC) and the parietal cortex, during REM sleep. In contrast, there is overall reduced brain activity during non-REM sleep (Larson-Prior et al., 2014).

Circadian Rhythms

Zeitgebers: External Cues to Synchronize Circadian Rhythms

○ Light

○ Melatonin

○ Eating and Drinking Patterns

○ Social Interactions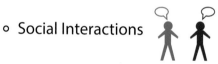

FIGURE 1.6. Virtually all living creatures have an internal molecular clock that synchronizes biological processes such as the sleep/wake cycle and metabolism to a 24-hour circadian rhythm. Although the molecular clock is self-sustaining, it needs to be reset daily. If the molecular clock is not reset, it will drift and become out of sync with environmental cues. These synchronizing cues, termed zeitgebers, include light/dark cycles generated by the movement of the Earth, endogenous or exogenous melatonin, social interactions, and food availability (Van Someren et al., 2007).

Light: The Most Powerful Zeitgeber

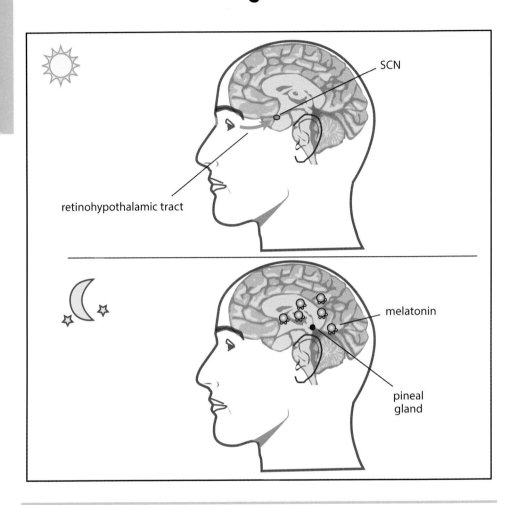

FIGURE 1.7. Although various factors can reset the clock, light is the most powerful synchronizer. When light enters through the eye, it is transferred via the retinohypothalamic tract to the suprachiasmatic nucleus (SCN) within the hypothalamus. During periods of darkness, the SCN induces the release of melatonin from the pineal gland, whereas light suppresses the release of melatonin (Zawilska, 2009).

Control of Sleep by the Suprachiasmatic Nucleus

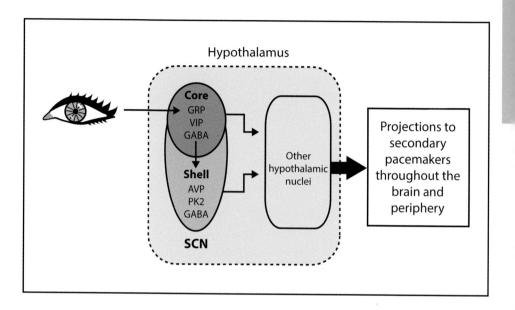

FIGURE 1.8. The main circadian pacemaker is the suprachiasmatic nucleus (SCN), which is located in the hypothalamus. The hypothalamus coordinates the secondary oscillators that are located throughout the periphery and that control many physiological functions, including metabolism, hormone secretion, and cell division. The SCN consists of 2 primary subregions: a ventrolateral core and a dorsomedial shell. The core contains neurons that release the neuropeptides vasoactive intestinal peptide (VIP) and gastrin-releasing peptide (GRP) as well as the neurotransmitter GABA. The core receives the majority of the light coming through the retinohypothalamic tract (as well as input from other brain regions) and utilizes this information to synchronize the SCN with light/dark cycles. The shell of the SCN contains neurons that release arginine vasopressin (AVP), prokineticin 2 (PK2), and GABA. These neurons receive input from the SCN core and use this information to synchronize the SCN with peripheral oscillators (Brancaccio et al., 2014; Colwell, 2011).

Brain Regions Involved in the Sleep/Wake Cycle

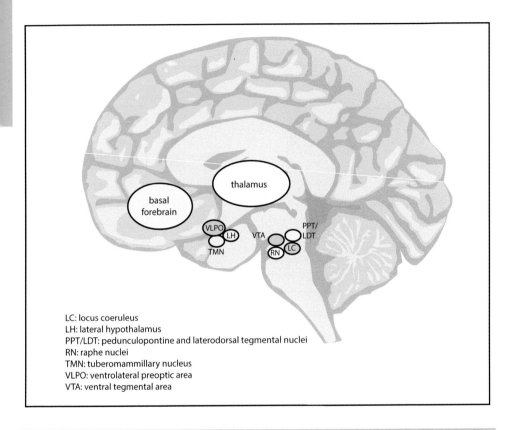

LC: locus coeruleus
LH: lateral hypothalamus
PPT/LDT: pedunculopontine and laterodorsal tegmental nuclei
RN: raphe nuclei
TMN: tuberomammillary nucleus
VLPO: ventrolateral preoptic area
VTA: ventral tegmental area

FIGURE 1.9. The sleep/wake cycle is maintained by a series of sleep-promoting and wake-promoting circuits located throughout the brain. Utilizing a variety of neurotransmitter and neuropeptide molecules, these circuits modulate one another via an intricate series of interacting loops (Roth and Roehrs, 2000).

The Sleep Circuit

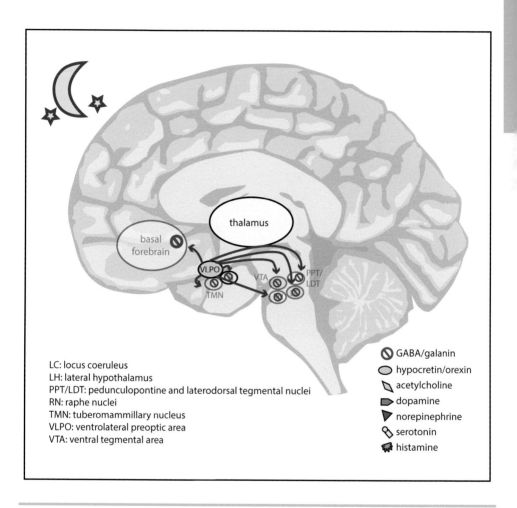

FIGURE 1.10. The sleep circuit is dependent upon the release of GABA and galanin from the ventrolateral preoptic (VLPO) nucleus of the hypothalamus. During periods of darkness, GABAergic projections from the VLPO area inhibit activity in brain regions of the wake-promoting circuit, including the tuberomammillary nucleus (TMN), the lateral hypothalamus (LH), the basal forebrain (BF), the pedunculopontine and laterodorsal tegmental (PPT/LDT) nuclei, the ventral tegmental area (VTA), the locus coeruleus (LC), and the raphe nuclei (RN).

The Wake Circuit: Part 1

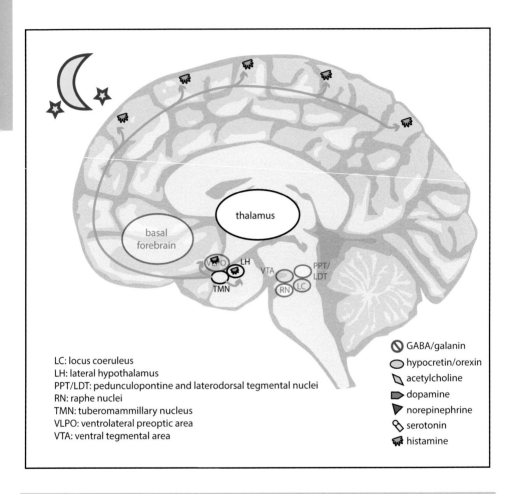

LC: locus coeruleus
LH: lateral hypothalamus
PPT/LDT: pedunculopontine and laterodorsal tegmental nuclei
RN: raphe nuclei
TMN: tuberomammillary nucleus
VLPO: ventrolateral preoptic area
VTA: ventral tegmental area

GABA/galanin
hypocretin/orexin
acetylcholine
dopamine
norepinephrine
serotonin
histamine

FIGURE 1.11. During periods of light, histamine is released from the tuberomammillary nucleus onto neurons throughout the cortex and in the ventrolateral preoptic area, inhibiting the release of GABA.

The Wake Circuit: Part 2

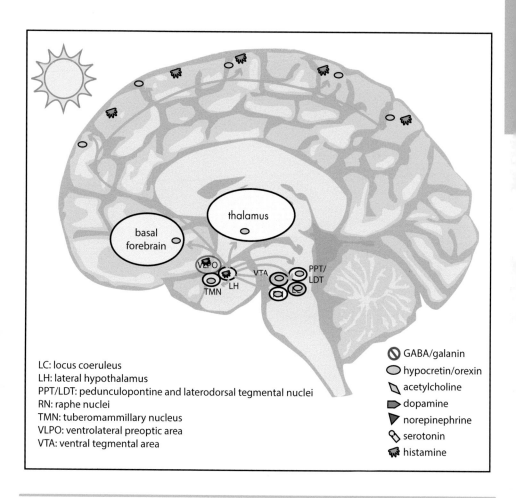

basal forebrain

thalamus

VLPO
TMN
LH
VTA
PPT/LDT

LC: locus coeruleus
LH: lateral hypothalamus
PPT/LDT: pedunculopontine and laterodorsal tegmental nuclei
RN: raphe nuclei
TMN: tuberomammillary nucleus
VLPO: ventrolateral preoptic area
VTA: ventral tegmental area

🚫 GABA/galanin
⬭ hypocretin/orexin
🗡 acetylcholine
▭ dopamine
▼ norepinephrine
🔑 serotonin
🦇 histamine

FIGURE 1.12. Histamine from the tuberomammillary nucleus also stimulates the release of hypocretin (also known as orexin) from the hypothalamus, specifically the lateral hypothalamus as well as the perifornical area and the posterior hypothalamus. There are 2 types of hypocretin/orexin molecules produced: orexin A and orexin B. The actions of these hypocretin/orexin molecules throughout the brain is believed to activate other elements of the wake-promoting circuit. In fact, it has been hypothesized that the hypocretin/orexin system may coordinate and maintain the activity of virtually all other components of the wake circuit (Stahl, 2013; Bonnavion and de Lecca, 2010).

The Wake Circuit: Part 3

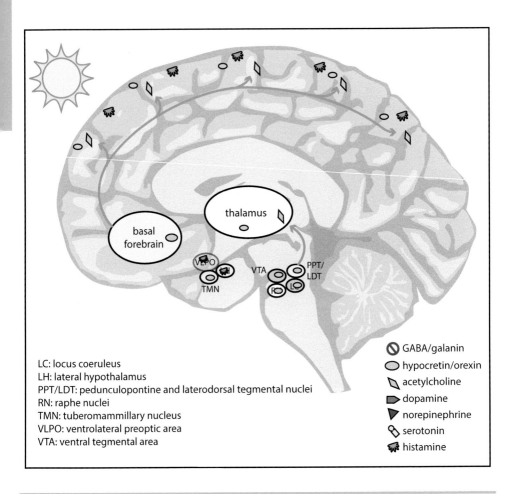

thalamus

basal forebrain

VLPO

VTA

PPT/LDT

TMN

LC: locus coeruleus
LH: lateral hypothalamus
PPT/LDT: pedunculopontine and laterodorsal tegmental nuclei
RN: raphe nuclei
TMN: tuberomammillary nucleus
VLPO: ventrolateral preoptic area
VTA: ventral tegmental area

GABA/galanin
hypocretin/orexin
acetylcholine
dopamine
norepinephrine
serotonin
histamine

FIGURE 1.13. Hypocretin/orexin induces the release of acetylcholine from the basal forebrain in cortical areas and the release of acetylcholine from the pedunculopontine and laterodorsal tegmental nuclei onto the thalamus.

The Wake Circuit: Part 4

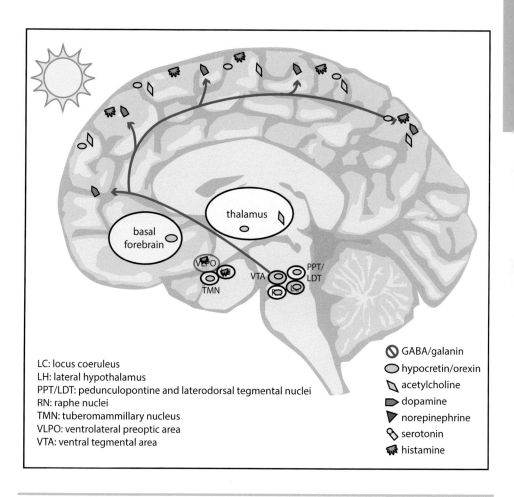

FIGURE 1.14. Hypocretin/orexin also causes the release of dopamine from the ventral tegmental area onto cortical areas.

The Wake Circuit: Part 5

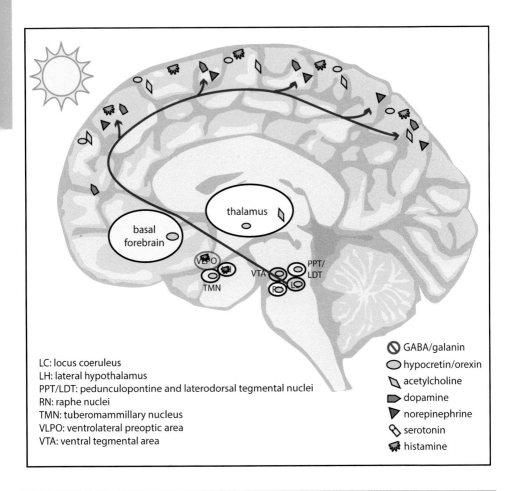

FIGURE 1.15. Additionally, hypocretin/orexin stimulates the release of norepinephrine from the locus coeruleus onto cortical areas.

The Wake Circuit: Part 6

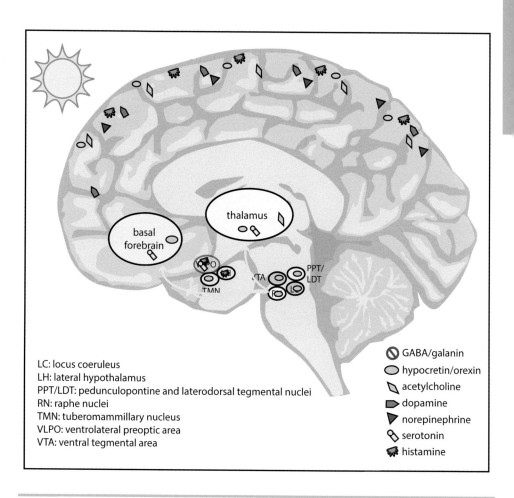

FIGURE 1.16. Hypocretin/orexin also instigates the release of serotonin from the raphe nuclei onto both the basal forebrain and the thalamus.

Triggering the Sleep Circuit

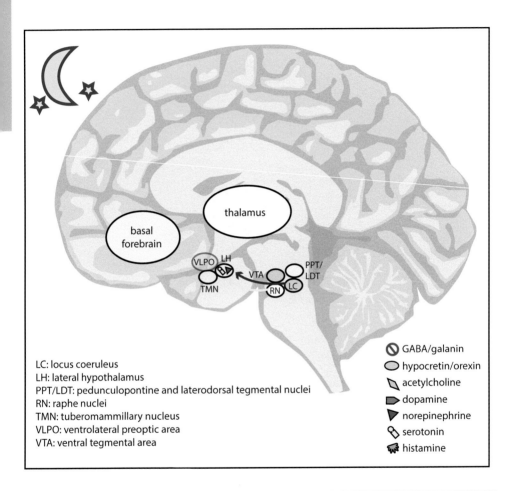

thalamus

basal forebrain

VLPO LH

VTA PPT/LDT

TMN

RN LC

LC: locus coeruleus
LH: lateral hypothalamus
PPT/LDT: pedunculopontine and laterodorsal tegmental nuclei
RN: raphe nuclei
TMN: tuberomammillary nucleus
VLPO: ventrolateral preoptic area
VTA: ventral tegmental area

GABA/galanin
hypocretin/orexin
acetylcholine
dopamine
norepinephrine
serotonin
histamine

FIGURE 1.17. Furthermore, norepinephrine from the locus coeruleus and serotonin from the raphe nuclei are released onto neurons in the lateral hypothalamus, inhibiting the release of hypocretin. Without hypocretin/orexin, the ventrolateral preoptic nucleus is disinhibited. The activated ventrolateral preoptic nucleus therefore releases GABA and galanin, inhibiting wake circuitry and initiating the sleep circuit.

Neurotransmitter Levels Throughout the Sleep/Wake Cycle: GABA/Galanin

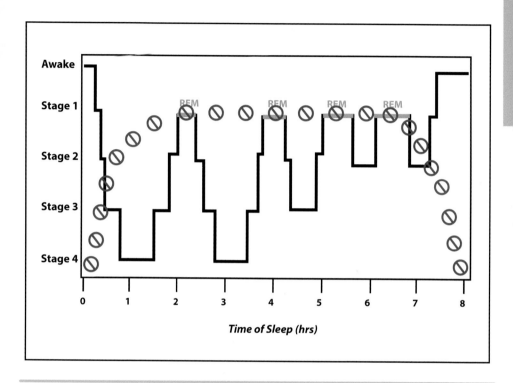

FIGURE 1.18. Neurotransmitters fluctuate not only on a circadian (24-hour) basis, but also throughout the sleep cycle. GABA and galanin levels steadily increase during the first couple of hours of sleep, plateau, and then steadily decline before one wakes.

Neurotransmitter Levels Throughout the Sleep/Wake Cycle: Hypocretin/Orexin

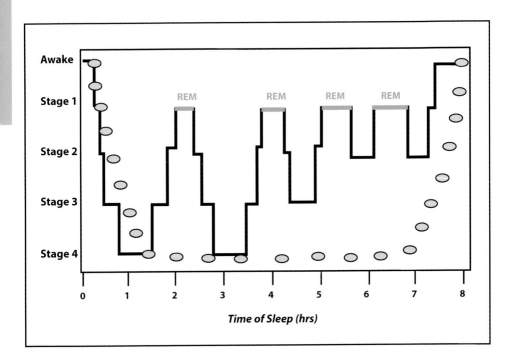

FIGURE 1.19. Unlike GABA/galanin levels, hypocretin/orexin levels steadily decrease during the first couple of hours of sleep, plateau, and then steadily increase before one wakes.

Neurotransmitter Levels Throughout the Sleep/Wake Cycle: Acetylcholine

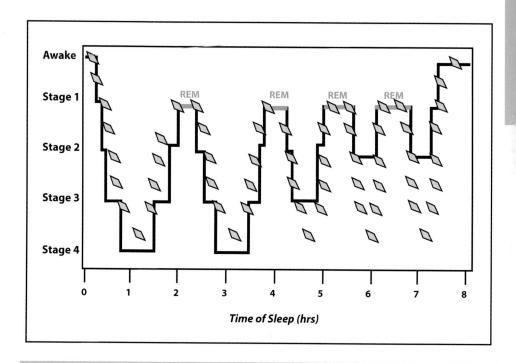

FIGURE 1.20. Acetylcholine levels fluctuate throughout the sleep cycle, reaching their lowest levels during stage 4 sleep and peaking during REM sleep.

Neurotransmitter Levels Throughout the Sleep/Wake Cycle: Dopamine, Norepinephrine, Serotonin, and Histamine

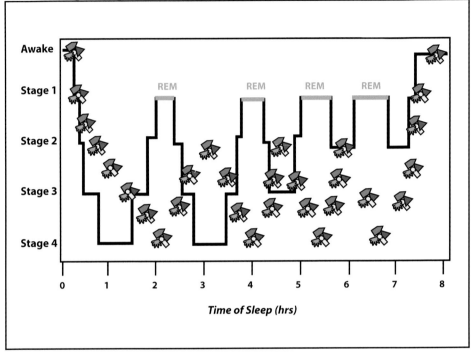

FIGURE 1.21. Dopamine, norepinephrine, serotonin, and histamine levels demonstrate a different trend. They peak during stage 2 sleep and are at their lowest during REM sleep.

Hypocretin/Orexin

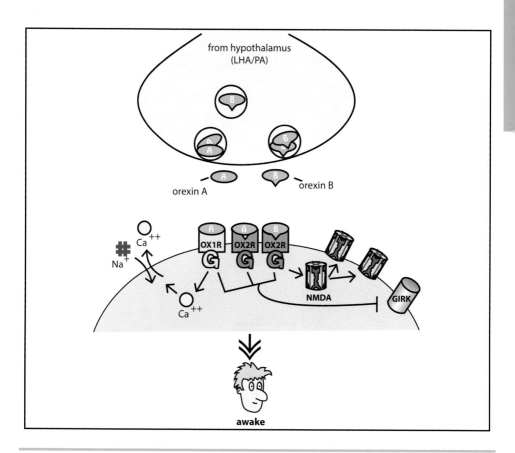

FIGURE 1.22. Hypocretin/orexin neurotransmission is mediated by 2 types of postsynaptic G-protein-coupled receptors: orexin 1 (Ox1R) and orexin 2 (Ox2R). The neurotransmitter orexin A is capable of interacting with both Ox1R and Ox2R, whereas the neurotransmitter orexin B binds selectively to Ox2R. The binding of orexin A to Ox1R leads to increased intracellular calcium as well as activation of the sodium/calcium exchanger. The binding of orexin A or B to Ox2R leads to increased expression of N-methyl-D-aspartate (NMDA) glutamate receptors as well as inactivation of G-protein-regulated inwardly rectifying potassium (GIRK) channels. Ox1R are highly expressed in the noradrenergic locus coeruleus, whereas Ox2R are highly expressed in the histaminergic tuberomammillary nucleus (TMN) (Stahl, 2013; de Lecca and Huerta, 2015; Jones and Hassani, 2013).

Hypocretin/Orexin Projections

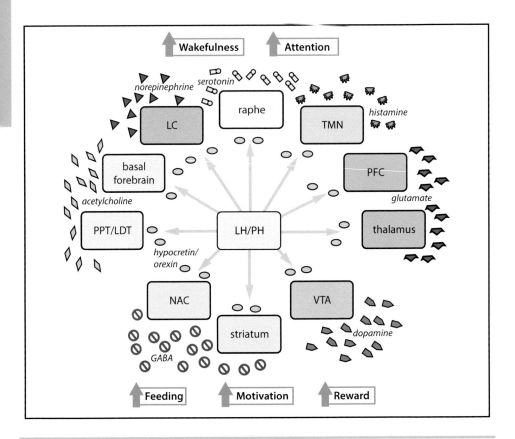

FIGURE 1.23. As previously discussed, hypocretin/orexin circuits originating from the hypothalamus project throughout the brain. These projections impart various effects depending on the target brain structure. For example, the following actions are hypothetically involved in maintaining wakefulness and attention: orexinergic stimulation of acetylcholine from the basal forebrain and the pedunculopontine and laterodorsal tegmental (PPT/LDT) nuclei, norepinephrine release from the locus coeruleus (LC), serotonin release from the raphe nuclei, histamine release from the tuberomammillary nucleus (TMN), and glutamate release from the prefrontal cortex (PFC) and the thalamus. Similarly, GABA release from the nucleus accumbens (NAC) and the striatum as well as dopamine release from the ventral tegmental area (VTA) are believed to be involved in feeding, motivation, and reward-directed behaviors (Scammel and Winrow, 2011).

Hypocretin/Orexin and Motivated Behaviors

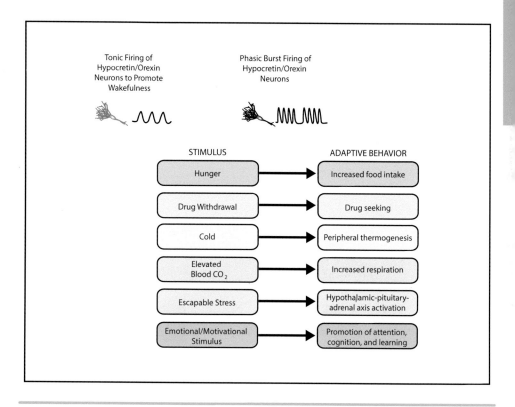

FIGURE 1.24. During periods of wakefulness, hypocretin/orexin neurons are active and fire with tonic frequency to maintain arousal. When presented with a stimulus—either external, such as an escapable stressor, or internal, such as elevated CO2 levels—hypocretin/orexin neurons exhibit a more rapid phasic burst firing pattern. This excitement of hypocretin/orexin neurons leads to increased neurotransmission and the activation of other brain areas and peripheral responses; in turn, this leads to the execution of appropriate behavioral responses. These behavioral responses lead to the attainment of reward or the avoidance of potential danger. In this way, the hypocretin/orexin system not only mediates wakefulness, but also allows for the facilitation of goal-directed, motivated behaviors, including increased food intake in response to hunger (Mahler et al., 2014).

Histamine

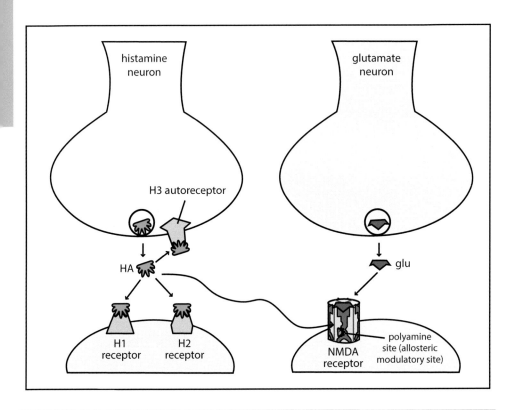

FIGURE 1.25. Shown here are receptors for histamine that regulate its neurotransmission. Histamine 1 and histamine 2 receptors are postsynaptic, while histamine 3 receptors are presynaptic autoreceptors. There is also a binding site for histamine on NMDA receptors; it can act at the polyamine site, which is an allosteric modulatory site (Stahl, 2013).

Melatonin

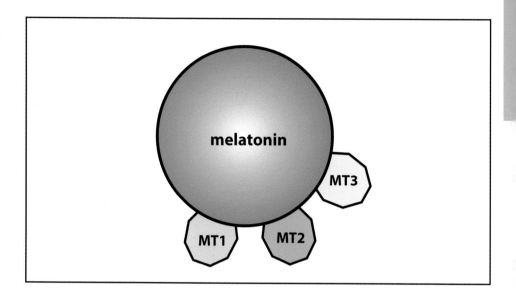

FIGURE 1.26. Endogenous melatonin is secreted by the pineal gland and mainly acts in the suprachiasmatic nucleus to regulate circadian rhythms. There are 3 types of receptors for melatonin: melatonin 1 and 2 (MT1 and MT2), which are both involved in sleep and circadian rhythms, and melatonin 3 (MT3), which is not thought to be involved in sleep physiology (Stahl, 2013).

The Molecular Clock: Transcription Factors

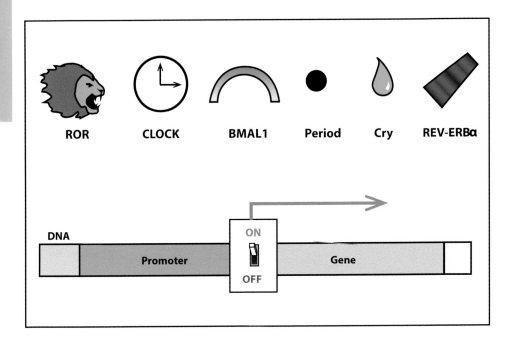

FIGURE 1.27. Behaviors that follow circadian rhythms, including sleep/wake patterns, are regulated at the molecular level by an intricate series of feedback loops that comprise the "molecular clock." Recent data indicate that disturbance of the molecular clock may be involved in various mental and physical illnesses (Froy, 2010; Green et al., 2008; Sahar and Sassone-Corsi, 2009; Takahashi et al., 2008; Arallanes-Licea et al., 2014; Banerjee et al., 2014; Brancaccio et al., 2014; Golombek et al., 2013; Qureshi and Mehler, 2014). The molecular clock consists of several transcription factors (i.e., proteins that bind to the promoter regions of DNA and in doing so, turn the expression of a gene on or off) that regulate each other's expression as well as the expression of many other genes involved in nearly all physiological processes. In fact, it has been estimated that as much as 10% of the genome is under the control of the CLOCK/BMAL1 complex (Masri et al., 2015).

The Molecular Clock

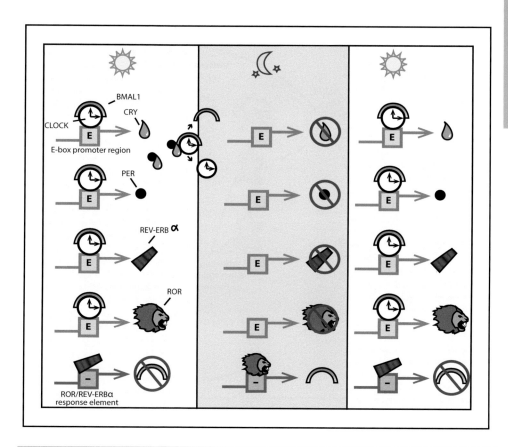

FIGURE 1.28. The proteins circadian locomotor output cycles kaput (CLOCK) and brain and muscle ARNT-like-1 (BMAL1) form a heterodimer that binds to E-box sequences in the promoter regions of numerous genes that are expressed in a circadian manner. Two such genes under the regulatory control of the CLOCK/BMAL1 complex are those that encode period (PER) and cryptochrome (CRY). Following their buildup during the day, PER and CRY form a complex that inhibits the actions of CLOCK/BMAL1. Another gene whose expression is controlled by CLOCK/BMAL1 is the one that encodes REV-ERBα. REV-ERBα is itself a transcription factor whose binding to the ROR/REV-ERBα response element (RRE) prevents the expression of the gene for BMAL1. The binding of retinoic acid-related orphan receptor (ROR) to the RRE has the opposite effect on BMAL1 expression; it leads to increased production of BMAL1 (Brancaccio et al., 2014; Cirelli, 2009).

Light Control of the Molecular Clock: Part 1

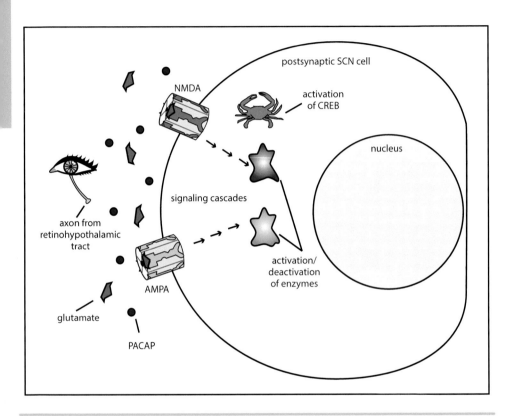

FIGURE 1.29. When light enters through the eye, it is translated via melanopsin-expressing retinal ganglion cells into action potentials that travel via the retinohypothalamic tract to the suprachiasmatic nucleus (SCN) within the hypothalamus. Within the SCN, glutamate, which acts on both NMDA and AMPA receptors, and the pituitary adenylate cyclase-activating polypeptide (PACAP), which enhances glutamate signaling, are released and increase the activity of neurons in the SCN. This increased activity of SCN neurons leads to an influx of Ca2+ and the subsequent activation of many intracellular signaling cascades. The downstream effects of these signaling cascades include the activation or deactivation of various enzymes that are responsible for maintaining or degrading functional molecular clock proteins as well as the activation of proteins that regulate the transcription and translation of molecular clock genes, including cyclic AMP response element binding protein (CREB) (Colwell, 2011).

Light Control of the Molecular Clock: Part 2

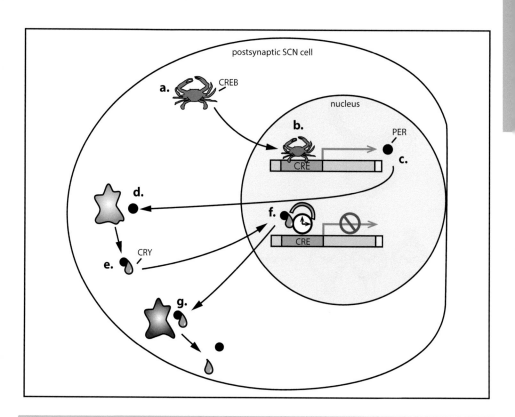

FIGURE 1.30. Photic activation of CREB and kinases is essential for maintaining the cycle of the molecular clock. For example, **a)** activated CREB may **b)** enter the nucleus and act on the CREB response element (CRE) found on the period (Per) gene, **c)** thus turning on the expression of Per (Colwell, 2011). **d)** When Per leaves the nucleus, **e)** it is joined with cryptochrome (Cry) to form a heterodimer that can enter the nucleus. **f)** Once inside the nucleus, the Per/Cry complex prevents CLOCK/BMAL1-induced expression of other components of the molecular clock as well as CLOCK/BMAL1-controlled expression of many genes involved in metabolism, cell cycle regulation, and virtually all physiological functions (Arallanes-Licea et al., 2014). **g)** Per and Cry proteins are degraded outside the nucleus, leading to the disinhibition of Clock/BMAL1-controlled gene expression and the initiation of a new 24-hour cycle (Brancaccio et al., 2014).

Misalignment Between Central and Peripheral Clocks

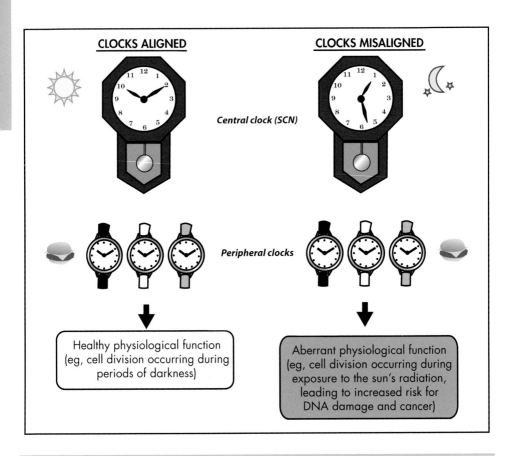

FIGURE 1.31. Food intake is able to efficiently entrain peripheral oscillators, such as those controlling metabolism, endocrine functions, and cell division, whereas the entrainment of the central pacemaker (i.e., the suprachiasmatic nucleus (SCN)) relies most heavily on light as its primary zeitgeber (Green et al., 2008). If the timing of the entrainment of the peripheral and central clocks becomes desynchronized—such as occurs with shift work disorder, in which patients eat during periods of darkness—this misalignment can have dire effects on a myriad of physiological functions. This misalignment may greatly increase one's risk of cardiometabolic disorders, endocrine dysfunction, and cancer (Oosterman et al., 2014).

Regulation of Neurotransmitters by the Molecular Clock

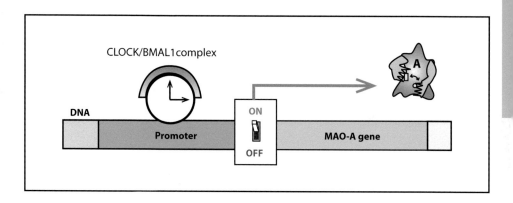

FIGURE 1.32. It is widely agreed that disturbances in neurotransmitter systems are the neurobiological basis of many psychiatric disorders. Interestingly, it has recently been determined that a gene for monoamine oxidase-A (MAO-A) is one of the many genes that are regulated by the CLOCK/BMAL1 complex and PER (Hampp et al., 2008). MAO-A is involved in the degradation of many neurotransmitters, including dopamine, norepinephrine, and serotonin. In fact, it has been shown that MAO-A is elevated in major depression, leading to decreased monoamines such as serotonin, and low in schizophrenia, leading to increased monoamines such as dopamine (Meyer et al., 2006). These data not only reinforce the use of pharmacological agents to modify neurotransmitter systems through receptor agonism or antagonism, but also support the use of nonpharmacological agents, such as light therapy, and pharmacological agents that may modify circadian rhythms.

Sleep and Psychiatry

Clock Genes Associated With Psychiatric Disorders		
Clock Gene	**Disorder**	**References**
BMAL	Bipolar disorder	Mansour et al. 2006; Nievergelt et al. 2006.
Clock (or its homolog, NPAS)	Bipolar disorder	Benedetti et al. 2003; Soria et al. 2010.
	Depression	Soria et al. 2010.
	Schizophrenia	Takao et al. 2007.
	Seasonal affective disorder	Johansson et al. 2003; Partonen et al. 2007.
Cry	Depression	Soria et al. 2010.
Per	Bipolar disorder	Nievergelt et al. 2006; Artioli et al. 2007; Mansour et al. 2006.
	Depression	Artioli et al. 2007.
	Schizophrenia	Mansour et al. 2006.
	Seasonal affective disorder	Partonen et al. 2007.
REV-ERBα	Bipolar disorder	Kripke et al. 2009; Severino et al. 2009.

FIGURE 1.33. Many individuals who suffer from psychiatric disorders have concurrent disturbances in sleep. In fact, particular sleep/wake patterns are often used in the diagnosis of many psychiatric disorders. The elimination of sleep disturbances may be essential for optimizing the treatment of mental illnesses; for example, the elimination of sleep disturbances in patients with depression alleviates depressive symptoms in up to 60% of cases (Orzel-Gryglewska, 2010). It is therefore not surprising that polymorphisms in the genes for BMAL, CLOCK, Cry, Per, and REV-ERB alpha have all been associated with various psychiatric disorders, including bipolar disorder, depression, schizophrenia, and seasonal affective disorder.

Sleep and Cognition

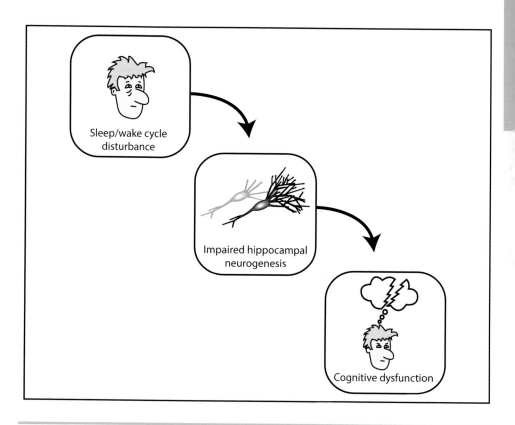

Sleep/wake cycle disturbance

Impaired hippocampal neurogenesis

Cognitive dysfunction

FIGURE 1.34. Disturbances in the sleep/wake cycle can have profound effects on cognitive functioning, including impairments in attention, memory deficits, and an inability to process new information. In fact, 24 hours of sleep deprivation or chronic short sleep duration (i.e., 4-5 hours/night) results in cognitive impairments equivalent to those seen with a 1% blood alcohol intoxication (Orzel-Gryglewska, 2010). Both REM and non-REM sleep appear to be essential for optimal cognitive functioning, with REM sleep modulating affective memory consolidation and non-REM sleep being critical for declarative and procedural memory (Dresler et al., 2014). At the neurobiological level, there is evidence that disruption of the sleep/wake cycle impairs hippocampal neurogenesis, which may partly explain the behavioral effects of sleep/wake cycle disturbances on cognition (Golombek et al., 2013).

Circadian Rhythms and Cell Division

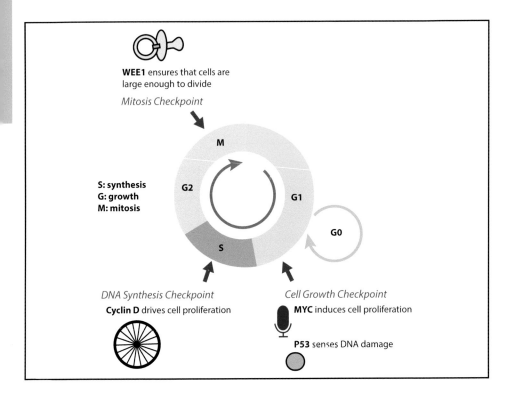

WEE1 ensures that cells are large enough to divide

Mitosis Checkpoint

M

S: synthesis
G: growth
M: mitosis

G2

G1

G0

S

DNA Synthesis Checkpoint
Cyclin D drives cell proliferation

Cell Growth Checkpoint
MYC induces cell proliferation

P53 senses DNA damage

FIGURE 1.35. There are several links between disturbed circadian function and cancer risk. Cell division is closely regulated by cell cycle genes, including WEE1, MYC, Cyclin D, and p53. These cell cycle genes oscillate with a circadian rhythm under at least partial control of the molecular clock. For example, the expression of WEE1 and MYC is regulated by the CLOCK/BMAL1 complex (Takahashi et al., 2008; Masri et al., 2015). If CLOCK/BMAL1 expression is dysregulated—for instance, due to misalignment between the central and peripheral clocks—WEE1 and MYC expression will also be disrupted, leading to increased cell division during daylight and consequent exposure to DNA-damaging ultraviolet radiation. Additionally, at least one of the molecular clock components, period (PER), has been shown to have tumor-suppressing capabilities; thus, aberrant expression of PER or even certain polymorphisms in the PER gene may increase one's risk for cancer (Sahar and Sassone-Corsi, 2009).

Cancer and Circadian Rhythms

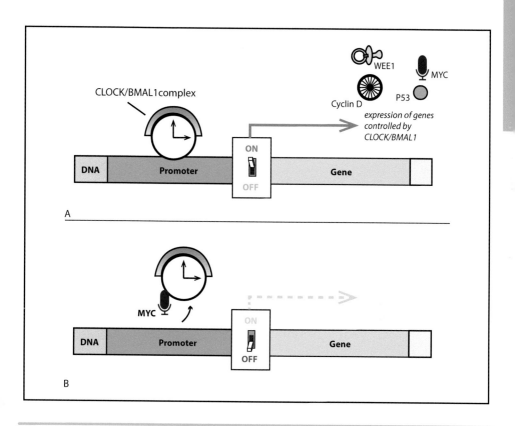

FIGURE 1.36. Cell division is regulated by the molecular clock, and aberrant cell division may regulate circadian rhythms. There is evidence that DNA damage may function as a zeitgeber, resetting the molecular clock (Sahar and Sassone-Corsi, 2009; Takahashi et al., 2008). As an example of this reciprocal relationship between cell division and the molecular clock, both MYC and p53 can prevent the binding of the CLOCK/BMAL1 complex to promoter regions, leading to the aberrant expression of many genes, including other components of the molecular clock, such as Per and Cry (Masri et al., 2015).

Sleep and Obesity

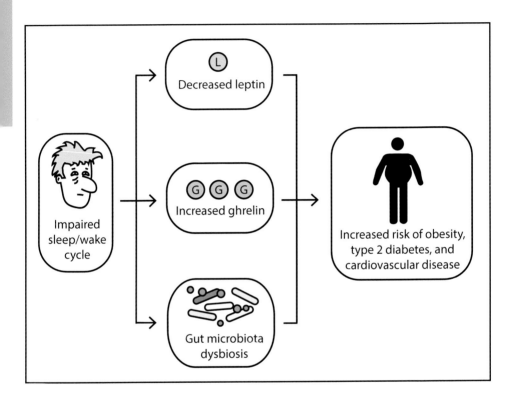

FIGURE 1.37. In recent years, much interest in the relationship between sleep and cardiometabolic issues such as type 2 diabetes and obesity has been expressed (Nixon et al., 2014). Although much remains unknown, an impaired sleep/wake cycle has been shown to disrupt the circulating levels of both the anorectic (appetite inhibiting) hormone leptin and the orexigenic (appetite stimulating) hormone ghrelin. These changes lead to dysfunctional insulin, glucose, and lipid metabolism; in turn, this may increase the risk of obesity, type 2 diabetes, and cardiovascular disease (Froy, 2010; Orzel-Gryglewska, 2010; Golombek et al., 2013). Additionally, an altered sleep/wake cycle has been shown to disturb the natural fluctuations in gut microbiota, perhaps further promoting glucose intolerance and obesity (Thaiss et al., 2014).

Nutrition and the Molecular Clock

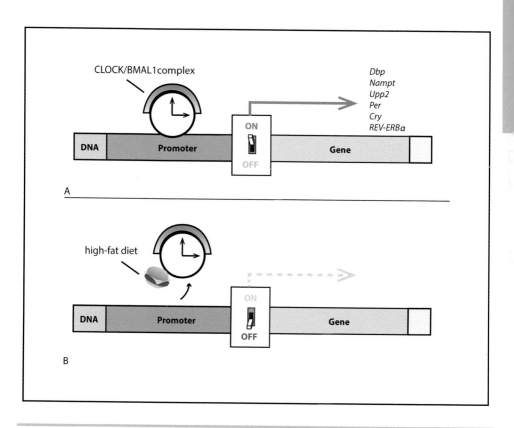

FIGURE 1.38. A high-fat diet prevents CLOCK/BMAL1 control of gene expression. A) The expression of many genes is regulated by the binding of the CLOCK/BMAL1 complex. Albumin D element-binding protein (Dbp), Per, Cry, and REV-ERBα are transcription factors involved in the regulation of the molecular clock and have various other functions. Nicotinamide phosphoribosyltransferase (Nampt) is involved in nicotinamide adenine dinucleotide (NAD+) synthesis and plays a role in many important biological processes, including metabolism, stress response, and aging. Uridine phosphorylase 2 (Upp2) is involved in metabolism and nucleotide synthesis. B) A high-fat diet prevents the CLOCK/BMAL1 complex from being recruited to DNA in its usual circadian manner. This leads to reduced and/or aberrant expression of Dbp, Per, Cry, REV-ERBα, Nampt, Upp2, and numerous other CLOCK/BMAL1-regulated genes and the consequent dysregulation of many physiological functions (Eckel-Mahan et al., 2013).

Sleep and Immunity

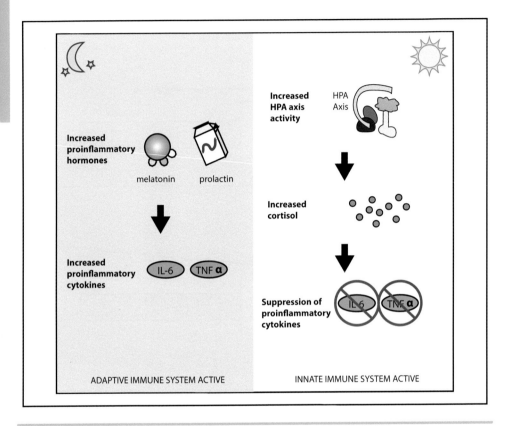

FIGURE 1.39. There are many associations between the sleep/wake cycle and immunity. During the night, there is an increased release of proinflammatory hormones such as prolactin and melatonin, an increased release of proinflammatory cytokines such as IL-6 and TNF alpha, and increased activity in cells of the adaptive (antigen-specific) immune system (i.e., B- and T-lymphocytes). In contrast, daytime brings about increased activity of the hypothalamic-pituitary-adrenal (HPA) axis, increased cortisol release, the suppression of proinflammatory cytokines and allergic reactions, and increased activity of the innate (non-antigen-specific) immune system (i.e., granulocytes, monocytes, and natural killer (NK) cells) (Cermakian et al., 2013). When the sleep/wake cycle is disrupted, this circadian function of the immune system is altered and may lead to immunodeficiency—and, consequently, decreased tumor surveillance—as well as systemic inflammation (Dresler et al., 2104; Golombek et al., 2013).

Autoimmunity in Disorders of Hypersomnolence

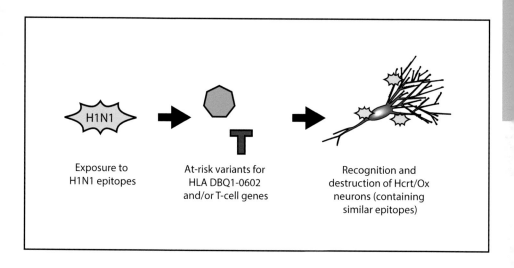

Exposure to H1N1 epitopes

At-risk variants for HLA DBQ1-0602 and/or T-cell genes

Recognition and destruction of Hcrt/Ox neurons (containing similar epitopes)

FIGURE 1.40. Both genetic and epidemiological data indicate that the profound loss of hypocretin/orexin (Hcrt/Ox) neurons seen in narcolepsy with cataplexy may be caused by an autoimmune reaction. An increase in the risk of developing narcolepsy has been seen following infection with the H1N1 influenza as well as the H1N1 vaccine (De la Herran-Arita and Garcia-Garcia, 2014). Additionally, genetic studies have shown a strong relationship between narcolepsy and polymorphisms in 2 key components of the immune system: the human leukocyte antigen (HLA) DBQ1-0602 gene and the T-cell receptor alpha gene (Sehgal and Mignot, 2011). It is therefore hypothesized that environmental exposure to certain antigens that are processed by HLA proteins (e.g., H1N1 influenza epitopes) leads to the activation of T-cells and may cause an autoimmune reaction that results in the destruction of Hcrt/Ox neurons in genetically predisposed individuals.

Assessment of Sleep/Wake Disorders

There are numerous, often co-occuring causes of both hypersomnia and hyposomnia. Optimizing patient outcomes relies on accurately identifying the neurobiological and behavioral causes of sleep/wake disturbances. In Chapter 2, we discuss the diagnostic tools available for assessing the degree of hyper- and hyposomnia as well as strategies for determining the etiology of excessive sleepiness or wakefulness.

Tools for Assessing Sleep/Wake Disorders: Polysomnography

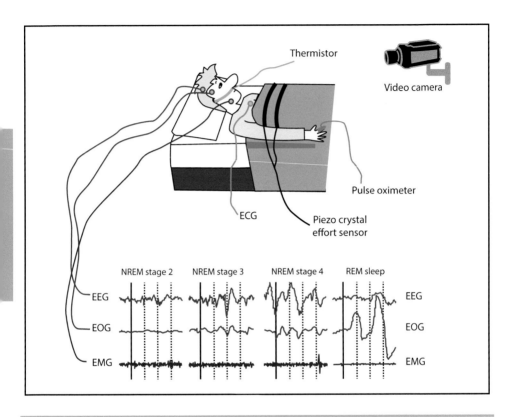

FIGURE 2.1. During polysomnography, an electroencephalogram (EEG) determines sleep stages; an electrooculogram (EOG) measures eye movement to identify rapid eye movement (REM) sleep; and an electromyogram (EMG) measures muscle activity via electrodes on the chin, jaw bone, and calf muscles. In addition, an electrocardiogram (ECG) is used to measure heart rate and rhythm, and breathing is measured with a piezo crystal effort sensor, which utilizes 2 Velcro bands around the chest and abdomen to measure movements and effort. Airflow is measured with a thermistor secured under the nose, and oxygen saturation can be measured by a pulse oximeter on the finger or ear lobe. Finally, the patient may be videotaped (Stahl, 2013).

Tools for Assessing Sleep/Wake Disorders: Multiple Sleep Latency Test

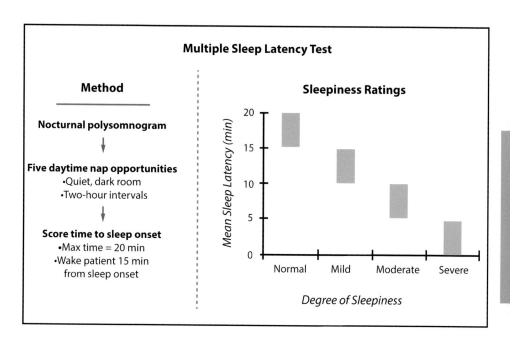

FIGURE 2.2. The Multiple Sleep Latency Test (MSLT) is a commonly used method for diagnosing sleep disorders. The test requires polysomnography equipment and must be performed by trained physicians in an accredited sleep lab. The degree of sleepiness is measured as the latency to the onset of any stage of sleep, with a mean latency of fewer than 10 minutes usually indicating excessive sleepiness related to a sleep disorder. However, there is some debate as to the actual MSLT threshold, with some experts supporting a cutoff of ⊠8 minutes to indicate excessive sleepiness (Plante, 2016). The Maintenance of Wakefulness Test is a similar test in which the patient is instructed to try to stay awake rather than try to fall asleep, as in the MSLT. Because there are different mechanisms for arousal maintenance and sleep induction, these tests can measure different aspects of excessive sleepiness (Sangal et al., 1992).

Tools for Assessing Sleep/Wake Disorders: Actigraphy

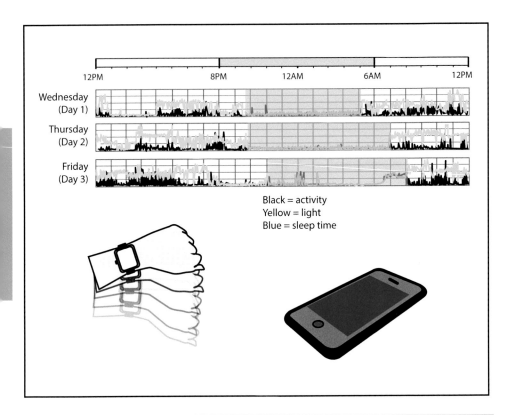

FIGURE 2.3. Actigraphy is used to record body movement over time in order to help assess sleep/wake patterns, including total sleep time and wake after sleep onset (WASO). Actigraphs are available as lightweight devices that can be worn on the wrist; they not only record movement, but also sense light (Martin and Hakim, 2011). There are now several smartphone apps available that can assess not only movement, but also noises, including snoring. At this time, these apps are not quite as accurate as laboratory measures; however, they are useful tools for in-home monitoring of sleep/wake and circadian rhythm issues as well as treatment effectiveness (Stippig et al., 2015).

Tools for Assessing Sleep/Wake Disorders: Sleep/Wake Diary

	Today's date (include month/day/year)	MON*	TUES	WED	THURS	FRI	SAT	SUN
COMPLETE IN MORNING	Time I went to bed last night Time I woke up this morning # of hours slept last night	11 pm 7am 8 hours						
	Number of awakenings and total time awake last night	5 times 2 hours						
	How long I took to fall asleep last night:	30 min.						
	How awake did I feel when I got up this morning? 1 = wide awake 2 = awake but a little tired 3 = sleepy	2						
COMPLETE IN EVENING	Number of caffeinated drinks (coffee, tea, cola) and time when I had them today:	1 drink at 8 pm						
	Number of alcoholic drinks (beer, wine, liquor) and time when I had them today:	2 drinks at 9 pm						
	Naptimes and lengths today:	3:30 pm for 45 min.						
	Exercise times and lengths today	30 min.						
	How sleep I felt during the day today: 1 = so sleepy I had to struggle to stay awake during much of the day 2 = somewhat tired 3 = fairly alert 4 = wide awake	1						
	*Example diary entries							

NAME:

FIGURE 2.4. Having patients keep a sleep/wake diary for 1–2 weeks can be very useful in assessing the contribution of poor sleep hygiene or medication use to sleep/wake or circadian rhythm problems.

Tools for Assessing Sleep/Wake Disorders: Epworth Sleepiness Scale

THE EPWORTH SLEEPINESS SCALE

How likely are you to doze off or fall asleep in the following situations, in contrast to just feeling tired? This refers to your usual way of life in recent times. Even if you have not done some of these things recently, try to work out how they each would have affected you. Use the following scale to choose the most appropriate number for each situation:

0 = Would never doze   2 = Moderate chance of dozing
1 = Slight chance of dozing   3 = High chance of dozing

Situation

Sitting and reading   _____

Watching TV   _____

Sitting, inactive in a public place (eg, a theater or a meeting)   _____

As a passenger in a car for an hour without a break   _____

Lying down to rest in the afternoon when circumstances permit   _____

Sitting and talking to someone   _____

Sitting quietly after a lunch without alcohol   _____

In a car, while stopped for a few minutes in traffic   _____

FIGURE 2.5. The Epworth Sleepiness Scale (ESS) is a self-rated, subjective measure of sleepiness. It is useful as a point-of-care tool for rapidly assessing the severity of sleepiness in a patient. For the general population, the average score on the ESS is approximately 5.9; a score over 10 indicates excessive sleepiness (Stahl, 2013).

Tools for Assessing Sleep/Wake Disorders: Pittsburgh Sleep Quality Index

During the past month, how often have you had trouble sleeping because you:				
	Not during the past month	Less than once a week	1-2 times a week	3+ times a week
a) Cannot get to sleep within 30 minutes				
b) Wake up in the middle of the night or early morning				
c) Have to get up to use the bathroom				
d) Cannot breathe comfortably				
e) Cough or snore loudly				
f) Feel too cold				
g) Feel too hot				
h) Had bad dreams				
i) Have pain				

FIGURE 2.6. The Pittsburgh Sleep Quality Index (PSQI) provides a self-reported measure of sleep quality and is useful for assessing insomnia (Buysse et al., 1989). The full PSQI as well as the scoring algorithm can be found at http://www.sleep. pitt.edu.

Tools for Assessing Sleep/Wake Disorders: Morningness-Eveningness Questionnaire

---

SAMPLE QUESTIONS INCLUDED IN THE MEQ

- Approximately what time would you get up if you were entirely free to plan your day?

- Approximately what time would you go to bed if you were entirely free to plan your evening?

- If you usually have to get up at a specific time in the morning, how much do you depend on an alarm clock?

- How easy do you find it to get up in the morning (when you are not awakened unexpectedly)?

- How alert do you feel during the first half hour after you wake up in the morning?

- How hungry do you feel during the first half hour after you wake up?

- During the first half hour after you wake up in the morning, how do you feel?

- If you had no commitments the next day, what time would you go to bed compared to your usual bedtime?

FIGURE 2.7. The Morningness-Eveningness Questionnaire (MEQ) is a useful assessment tool for determining an individual's "chronotype" (i.e., their natural circadian rhythm in terms of their sleep/wake cycle). The MEQ consists of 19 questions relating to when an individual would prefer to be awake or asleep (Horne and Östberg, 1976). An automated version of the MEQ (AutoMEQ) that includes estimated time for melatonin onset and "natural" bedtime as well suggested timing for bright light therapy can be found at http://www.cet.org/self-assessment/.

Commonly Used Psychotropics
That May Affect Sleep and Waking

Drug Type	Pharmacological Effect	Neurobiological Mechanism	Clinical Effects
SSRIs	Increase 5HT	5HT inhibits REM sleep	Decreased REM sleep
TCAs	Increase 5HT and NE	5HT and NE inhibit REM	Decreased REM sleep
Traditional amphetamine-like stimulants	Increase DA and NE	Increased DA and NE signaling	Increased wakefulness
Wake-promoting, nontraditional stimulants	Increase DA	Increased DA signaling	Increased wakefulness
Benzodiazepines	Enhance GABA signaling GABA-A receptors	GABA inhibits the arousal systems	Increased sleep
Nonbenzodiazepine sedatives	Enhance GABA signaling GABA-A receptors	GABA inhibits the arousal systems	Increased sleep
Antihistamines	Block HA H1 receptors	Reduced HA signaling	Increased sleep
Typical antipsychotics	Block DA receptors	Reduced DA signaling	Increased sleep

FIGURE 2.8. Many psychotropic agents impact the neurotransmitter systems that are involved in sleep/wake circuitry (discussed in Chapter 1). Therefore, when assessing sleep/wake disorders, it is important to determine if currently used medications may be contributing to disturbances in sleep/wake parameters. Many of these agents are also used in the treatment of sleep/wake disorders due to their ability to promote sleep or wakefulness (Espana and Scammell, 2011).

Insomnia: Excessive Nighttime Arousal

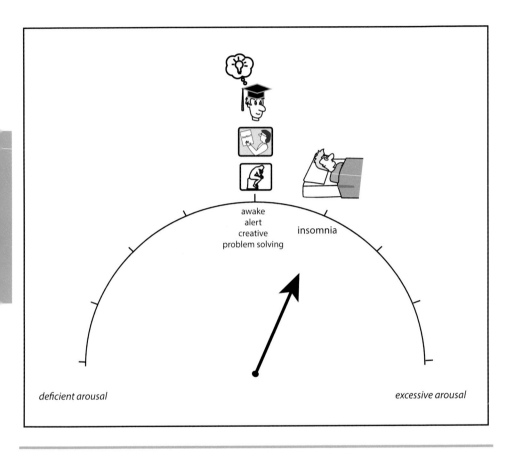

FIGURE 2.9. Insomnia is conceptualized as being related to hyperarousal at night, (Stahl, 2013).

Conditions Associated With Insomnia

Medical Conditions

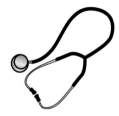

Substance Abuse

Psychiatric Conditions

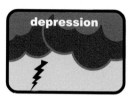

Behavioral/ Psychological Causes

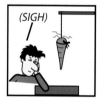

Medication Side Effects

Sleep/Wake Disorders

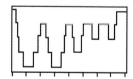

FIGURE 2.10. Approximately 40 million individuals in the United States suffer from chronic insomnia, and an additional 20 million suffer from episodic insomnia. However, as many as 70% of individuals with insomnia may not report it to their clinician (Reeve and Bailes, 2010). There are many conditions associated with insomnia, including improper sleep hygiene; medical illness; other sleep/wake disorders, including circadian rhythm disorders, restless legs syndrome, and sleep apnea; effects from medications or substances of abuse; and psychiatric disorders (Pinto Jr. et al., 2010; Morin and Benca, 2012; Schutte-Rodin et al., 2008). Insomnia may be self-perpetuating in that repeated episodes of wakefulness in bed may become associated with anxiety and sleeplessness (Harris et al., 2012).

Biology of Insomnia

Neuroanatomical Abnormalities
- Reduced gray matter in left orbitofrontal cortex and hippocampus

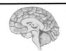

Neurobiological Abnormalities
- Decreased GABA levels in occipital and anterior cingulate cortices
- Reduced nocturnal melatonin secretion
- Increased glucose metabolism
- Attenuated sleep-related reduction in glucose metabolism in wake-promoting regions
- Decreased serum BDNF

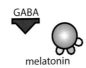

GABA

melatonin

BDNF

Autonomic Nervous System Abnormalities
- Heart rate elevations and variability
- Increased metabolic rate
- Increased body temp
- HPA axis activation
- Increased NE

HPA Axis

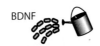

Systemic Inflammation

IL-6

Genetic Factors
- CLOCK gene polymorphisms
- GABA-A receptor gene polymorphisms
- Serotonin reuptake transporter (SERT) gene polymorphisms
- Human leukocyte antigen (HLA) gene polymorphisms
- Epigenetic modifications affecting genes involved in the response to stress

FIGURE 2.11. Several biological factors have been associated with insomnia, including increased activation of the autonomic nervous system, abnormal glucose metabolism, decreased GABA levels, reduced nocturnal melatonin secretion, systemic inflammation, and reduced brain volume (Morin and Benca, 2012; Krystal et al., 2013; Parthasarathy et al., 2015; Schutte-Rodin et al., 2008; Dresler et al., 2014). There are also several genetic factors that have been linked to an increased risk for insomnia (Palagini et al., 2014).

Insomnia and Psychiatric Illness

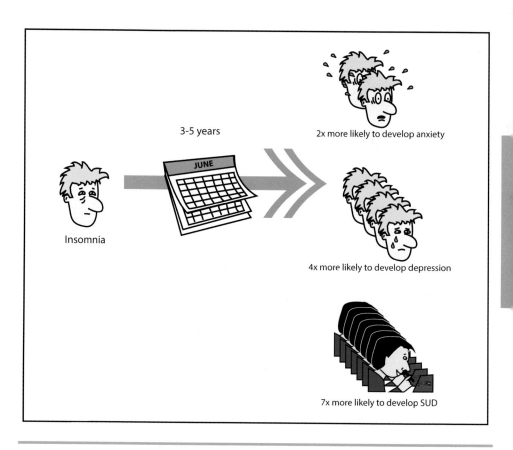

3-5 years

2x more likely to develop anxiety

JUNE

Insomnia

4x more likely to develop depression

7x more likely to develop SUD

FIGURE 2.12. Insomnia may be a risk factor for or a prodromal symptom of various psychiatric disorders, including depression, anxiety, and substance use disorders (Morin and Benca, 2012). Additionally, insomnia due to psychiatric illness, especially depression, may be more likely to persist than insomnia due to other causes (Vgontzas et al., 2012). Conversely, patients with depression who complain of insomnia (approximately 70% of individuals with depression) show worse treatment response, increased depressive episodes, and a worse overall long-term outcome (Dresler et al., 2014).

New DSM-5 Diagnostic Criteria for Insomnia

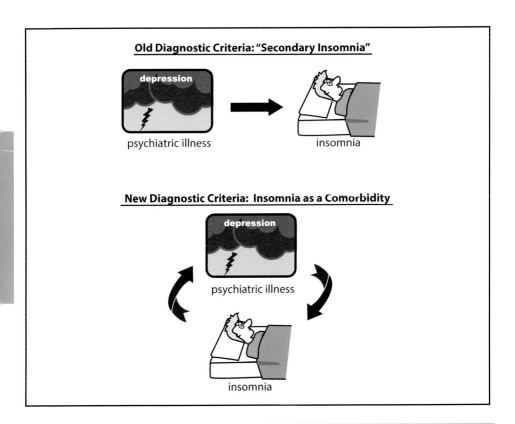

FIGURE 2.13. Insomnia has traditionally been categorized as either "secondary" (i.e., a symptom of a psychiatric or medical illness) or "primary" (i.e., neither associated with a psychiatric or medical illness nor a result of substance abuse or withdrawal) (Gupta et al., 2014). However, it is now more fully understood that insomnia is often a comorbidity rather than a symptom of psychiatric and medical illnesses. The newly revised DSM-5 diagnostic criteria for insomnia seek to do away with the concepts of secondary and primary insomnia and instead recognize the intricate 2-way, perpetuating relationship between insomnia and psychiatric and medical conditions.

Diagnosing Insomnia

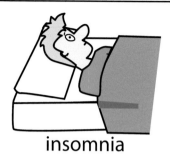

insomnia

Suggested criteria for defining insomnia:
Average sleep latency > 30 min
Wakefulness after sleep onset (WASO) > 30 min
Sleep efficiency < 85%
Total sleep time < 6.5 hours

FIGURE 2.14. Patients with insomnia often complain of poor sleep quality or duration, difficulty falling asleep, nighttime awakenings, or wake times that are earlier than desired (Morin and Benca, 2012). Many patients also report daytime fatigue, cognitive impairments, and mood disturbances (Schutte-Rodin et al., 2008). Polysomnography is not generally indicated for the diagnosis of insomnia but may be useful for ruling out narcolepsy, restless legs syndrome (RLS), or obstructive sleep apnea (OSA). Administration of the Epworth Sleepiness Scale (ESS) and the Pittsburgh Sleep Quality Index (PSQI) as well as the maintenance of a sleep/wake diary for at least 2 weeks are indicated (Reeve and Bailes, 2010). Although these subjective measures of sleep duration may not accurately equate to objective measures of sleep duration, they may be important given that subjective short sleep duration is more strongly associated with persistent insomnia and may be more difficult to treat (Vgontzas et al., 2012). Actigraphy may be useful for assessing the patient's sleep/wake cycles. A physical exam should also be performed to assess for sleep apnea, cardiovascular illness, endocrine disorders, or gastrointestinal conditions (Schutte-Rodin et al., 2008).

Tools for Assessing Sleep/Wake Disorders: Insomnia Severity Index

Please rate the CURRENT (i.e., LAST 2 WEEKS) SEVERITY of your insomnia problem(s).					
Insomnia problem	**None**	**Mild**	**Moderate**	**Severe**	**Very Severe**
1. Difficulty falling asleep	0	1	2	3	4
2. Difficulty staying asleep	0	1	2	3	4
3. Problem waking up too early	0	1	2	3	4

4. How SATISFIED/DISSATISFIED are you with your CURRENT sleep pattern?

Very Satisfied	**Satisfied**	**Moderately Satisfied**	**Dissatisfied**	**Very Dissatisfied**
0	1	2	3	4

5. How NOTICEABLE to others do you think your sleep problem is in terms of impairing the quality of your life?

Not at all Noticeable	**A Little**	**Somewhat**	**Much**	**Very much Noticeable**
0	1	2	3	4

6. How WORRIED/DISTRESSED are you about your current sleep problem?

Not at all Worried	**A Little**	**Somewhat**	**Much**	**Very Much Worried**
0	1	2	3	4

7. To what extent do you consider your sleep problem to INTERFERE with your daily functioning (e.g., daytime fatigue, mood, ability to function at work/daily chores, concentration, memory, mood) CURRENTLY?

Not at all Interfering	**A Little**	**Somewhat**	**Much**	**Very Much Interfering**
0	1	2	3	4

Total score categories:
0–7 = No clinically significant insomnia
8–14 = Subthreshold insomnia1
5–21 = Clinical insomnia (moderate severity)
22–28 = Clinical insomnia (severe)

FIGURE 2.15. The Insomnia Severity Index (ISI) is a 7-item, subjective questionnaire for assessing insomnia (Bastien et al., 2001).

Stahl's Illustrated

Excessive Daytime Sleepiness: Deficient Daytime Arousal?

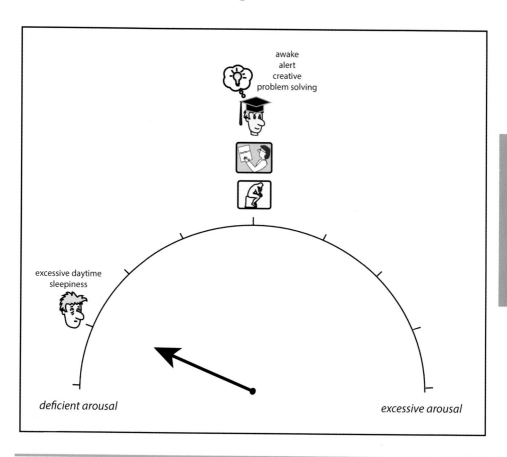

FIGURE 2.16. Excessive sleepiness is conceptualized as being related to hypoarousal during the day (Stahl, 2013).

Hypersomnia

Central Disorders of Hypersomnolence

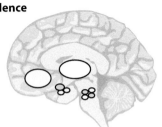

- Idiopathic hypersomnia
- Recurrent hypersomnia
- Narcolepsy with cataplexy
- Narcolepsy without cataplexy

Other Causes of Hypersomnia

- Medical conditions

- Medication side effects

- Substance abuse

- Psychiatric conditions

FIGURE 2.17. Hypersomnia is present in as much as 6% of the population (Dresler et al., 2014). Hypersomnia can occur in association with other sleep/wake disorders, medical conditions, medication side effects, or psychiatric illnesses (Adenuga and Attarian, 2014). In fact, as many as 25% of individuals with hypersomnia may have a mood disorder (Larson-Prior et al., 2014; Morgenthaler et al., 2007). There are also several disorders of hypersomnia that are not secondary to these other conditions and are thought to arise as a consequence of neuropathology in the sleep/wake circuitry of the brain. Such disorders are known as "central disorders of hypersomnolence" and include idiopathic hypersomnia, recurrent hypersomnia, and narcolepsy. With the exception of narcolepsy with cataplexy, the underlying neuropathology of the central disorders of hypersomnolence is largely unknown.

Idiopathic Hypersomnia

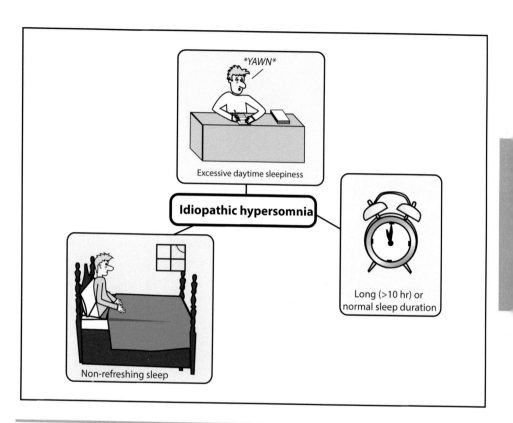

FIGURE 2.18. Idiopathic hypersomnia is characterized by either long or normal sleep duration accompanied by constant excessive daytime sleepiness, short sleep onset latency, and complaints of non-refreshing sleep. Patients with idiopathic hypersomnia may also report sleep drunkenness and somnolence following sleep. The diagnosis of idiopathic hypersomnia includes excessive daytime sleepiness lasting at least 3 months; a sleep latency of under 8 minutes, as determined by the Multiple Sleep Latency Test (MSLT); and fewer than 2 sleep onset REM periods (SOREMPs). Cerebrospinal fluid (CSF) levels of histamine may be low; however, unlike in narcolepsy with cataplexy, hypocretin levels are not typically affected (Dresler et al., 2014). Polysomnography should be performed to rule out other causes of hypersomnolence, and psychiatric and medical evaluations are also warranted, as idiopathic hypersomnia is often accompanied by memory and attention deficits, digestive system problems, depression, and anxiety (Larson-Prior et al., 2014; Morgenthaler et al., 2007).

Recurrent Hypersomnia

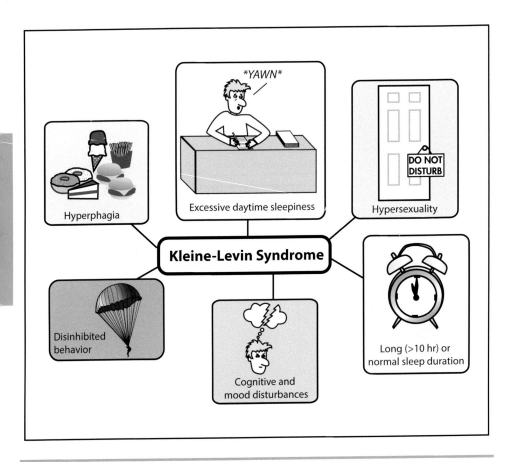

Hyperphagia

YAWN

Excessive daytime sleepiness

DO NOT DISTURB

Hypersexuality

Kleine-Levin Syndrome

Disinhibited behavior

Cognitive and mood disturbances

Long (>10 hr) or normal sleep duration

FIGURE 2.19. Recurrent hypersomnia is characterized by continuing excessive daytime sleepiness and may be associated with menstruation in women. However, Kleine-Levin syndrome is the most common form of recurrent hypersomnia. This rare disorder mostly affects adolescent boys and is characterized by bouts of hypersomnolence coupled with cognitive and mood disturbances, compulsive eating, hypersexuality, and disinhibited behavior (Dresler et al., 2014; Larson-Prior et al., 2014). Interestingly, accumulating data suggest an etiology of viral infection and subsequent autoimmune reaction, making Kleine-Levin syndrome similar to narcolepsy (Larson-Prior et al., 2014; Morgenthaler et al., 2007).

Narcolepsy

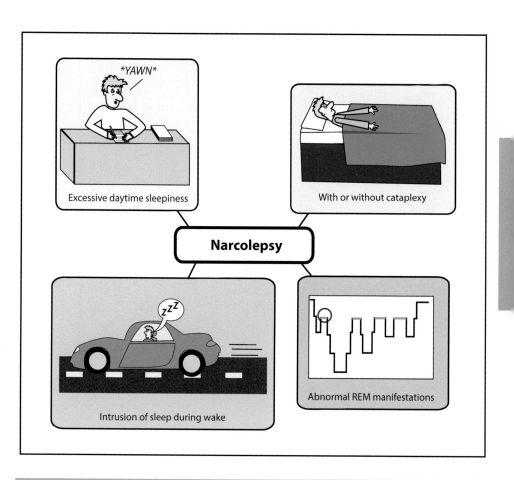

FIGURE 2.20. Narcolepsy is characterized by excessive daytime sleepiness, the intrusion of sleep during periods of wakefulness, and abnormal REM sleep, including periods of REM occurring at the onset of sleep (SOREMPs). Cataplexy, or loss of muscle tone triggered by emotions, may also be present. Hypnagogic hallucinations, which are present upon waking, are also often present (Adenuga and Attarian, 2014).

Neurobiology of Narcolepsy With Cataplexy

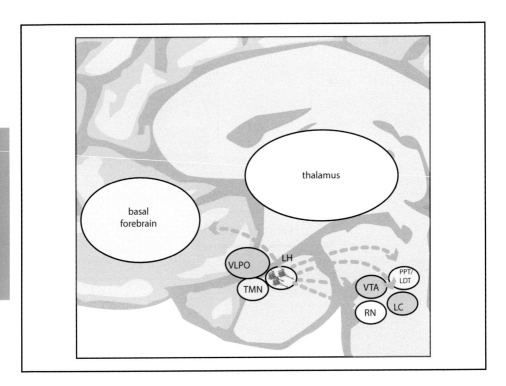

FIGURE 2.21. A clear neuropathological substrate has been identified for narcolepsy with cataplexy. Patients with narcolepsy with cataplexy exhibit a profound loss of hypocretin/orexin neurons in the lateral hypothalamus (LH). These neurons are involved in the maintenance of wakefulness through their actions on other components of the wake circuit. Additionally, the input of hypocretin/orexin neurons stimulates norepinephrine from the locus coeruleus (LC) and serotonin from the raphe nuclei (RN). The release of norepinephrine and serotonin influences the activation of motor neurons. During REM sleep, norepinephrine and serotonin activation of motor activity as well as components of the wake circuit are inhibited via GABA released from the ventrolateral preoptic nucleus (VLPO). Hypocretin/orexin normally prevents this inhibition of motor control during periods of wakefulness by turning off the VLPO. Given that hypocretin/orexin is necessary for the stabilization of wakefulness, it is not surprising that patients with loss of hypocretin/orexin neurons exhibit intrusion of sleep and cataplexy during periods of wakefulness (Adenuga and Attarian, 2014).

Differential Diagnosis of Hypersomnia

	Subjective Sleepiness	MSLT Sleep Latency	SOREMPs	Hcrt / Ox Levels
Narcolepsy with cataplexy	√	≤8 min.	≥2	Low ≤110 pg/mL
Narcolepsy without cataplexy	√	≤8 min.	≥2	Normal 200 - 700 pg/mL
Idiopathic hypersomnia	√	≤8 min.	<2	Normal 200 - 700 pg/mL
Recurrent hypersomnia	√ Episodic	Normal between episodes	<2	Normal 200 - 700 pg/mL

FIGURE 2.22. It is important to first eliminate and treat secondary causes of hypersomnia, such as obstructive sleep apnea, psychiatric illnesses, and medication side effects. This can be accomplished by conducting a full clinical interview, collecting data from a sleep/wake diary and 1–2 weeks' worth of actigraphy, performing polysomnography (PSG), and administering the Multiple Sleep Latency Test (MSLT) (Ahmed and Thorpy, 2010). A cerebrospinal fluid (CSF) hypocretin/orexin (Hcrt/Ox) level of <110 pg/mL is diagnostic for narcolepsy; however, Hcrt/Ox levels are often within normal range in narcolepsy, especially without cataplexy, as well as idiopathic and recurrent hypersomnia (Bourgin et al., 2008). Even in the absence of low Hcrt/Ox levels, patients with narcolepsy with or without cataplexy demonstrate ≥2 SOREMPs on the MSLT or 1 SOREMP on PSG as well as a short sleep latency (≤8 minutes) on the MSLT; thus, these measures are also considered diagnostic for narcolepsy (Dresler et al., 2014). Additionally, the majority (90%) of patients with narcolepsy, particularly those with cataplexy, are positive for the HLA DQB1-0602 polymorphism compared to only 20% of the general population (Mignot, 2012).

Circadian Rhythm Disorders

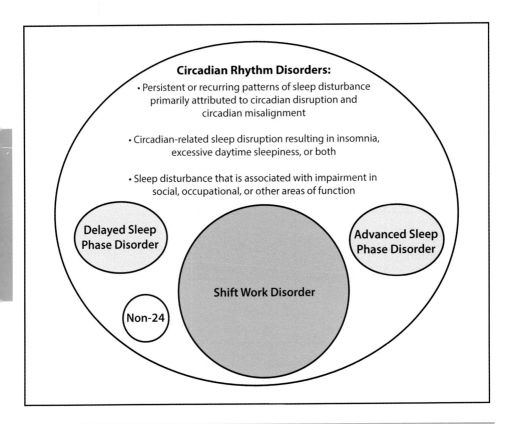

Circadian Rhythm Disorders:
- Persistent or recurring patterns of sleep disturbance primarily attributed to circadian disruption and circadian misalignment
- Circadian-related sleep disruption resulting in insomnia, excessive daytime sleepiness, or both
- Sleep disturbance that is associated with impairment in social, occupational, or other areas of function

Delayed Sleep Phase Disorder

Advanced Sleep Phase Disorder

Shift Work Disorder

Non-24

FIGURE 2.23. Circadian rhythm disorders arise when there is dyssynchrony between the internal clock and external cues that signal "daytime" and "nighttime." This dyssynchrony leads to difficulty maintaining a sleep/wake cycle within the typical 24-hour period. There are several circadian rhythm disorders, including shift work disorder, advanced sleep phase disorder, delayed sleep phase disorder, and Non-24-Hour Sleep-Wake disorder (Barger et al., 2012; Harrison and Gorman, 2012; Reeve and Bailes, 2010; Morgenthaler et al., 2007b).

Shift Work Disorder

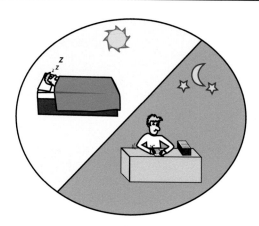

- Insomnia or excessive sleepiness temporarily associated with a recurring work schedule that overlaps with the usual time for sleep
- Symptoms associated with shift work schedule are present for at least 1 month
- Sleep log or actigraphy monitoring (with sleep diaries) for at least 7 days demonstrates disturbed sleep (insomnia) and circadian and sleep-time misalignment
- Sleep disturbance is not due to another current sleep disorder, medical disorder, mental disorder, substance use disorder, or medication use

FIGURE 2.24. Shift work is defined as work occurring between 6 pm and 7 am (outside the standard daytime working hours). Shift workers include those who work night shifts, evening shifts, or rotating shifts and comprise approximately 15-25% of the workforce in the United States. Shift workers' sleep/wake schedules are often out of sync with their endogenous circadian rhythms, and many (but not all) individuals who work non-standard or rotating schedules develop shift work disorder (SWD). In fact, it is estimated that as many as 10-32% of shift workers develop SWD and as many as 9.1% of shift workers develop a severe form of the disorder. Younger age and "eveningness" may provide some protection from the development of SWD. However, for those who do develop SWD, there may be physical and psychiatric consequences that extend far beyond sleep/wake disturbances, such as excessive sleepiness during the work shift and insomnia during periods of sleep. Individuals with SWD have a dramatically increased risk of cardiometabolic issues, cancer, gastrointestinal diseases, and mood disorders (Morrissette, 2013).

Advanced Sleep Phase Disorder

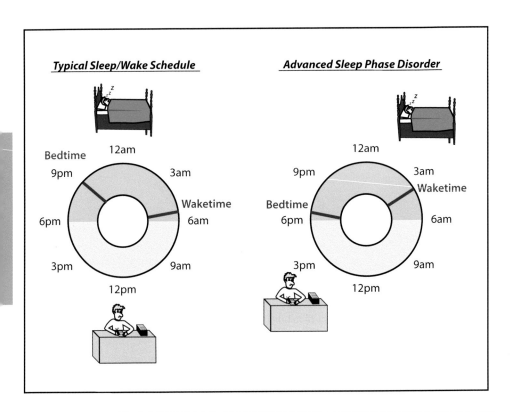

FIGURE 2.25. Although patients with advanced sleep phase disorder (ASPD) have adequate total sleep time and quality of sleep, they go to bed earlier and awaken earlier than desired, often by 4-6 hours outside of the typical sleep/wake cycle (Morgenthaler et al., 2007; Arallanes-Licea et al., 2014; Gupta et al., 2014). Polymorphisms in the PER2 gene (an essential component of the molecular clock discussed in Chapter 1) have been associated with ASPD; in fact, there is an autosomal dominant form of the disorder called familial advanced sleep phase syndrome (FASPS) in which a PER2 mutation is indicated (Takahashi et al., 2008; Golombek et al., 2013; Sehgal and Mignot, 2011; Tafti et al., 2007). In addition to ruling out other sleep/wake disorders, such as insomnia, diagnosing ASPD may include the use of a sleep diary and/or actigraphy for at least a week and the administration of the Morningness-Eveningness Questionnaire (MEQ). Treatments for ASPD include bright light therapy, chronobiotics (including melatonin, ramelteon, or tasimelteon), armodafinil/modafinil, and structured sleep/wake schedules.

Delayed Sleep Phase Disorder

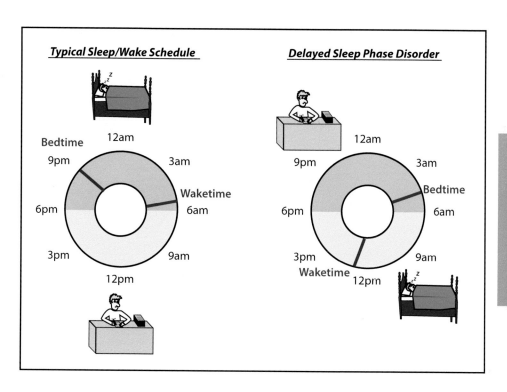

FIGURE 2.26. In delayed sleep phase disorder (DSPD), individuals are unable to fall asleep until early morning hours and awaken in the late morning/early afternoon (Morgenthaler et al., 2007). DSPD is the most common of the circadian rhythm disorders and has been associated with polymorphisms in the CLOCK gene (an essential element of the molecular clock discussed in Chapter 1) (Takahashi et al., 2008). Similar to advanced sleep phase disorder (ASPD), sleep duration and quality of sleep are normal; however, the shift in the sleep/wake schedule interferes with daily functioning (Gupta et al., 2014). Diagnosis and treatment of DSPD are similar to those of ASPD, with alterations to the timing of light or chronobiotic therapy administration (Golembek et al., 2013; Gupta et al., 2014; Morgenthaler et al., 2007).

Non-24-Hour Sleep-Wake Disorder

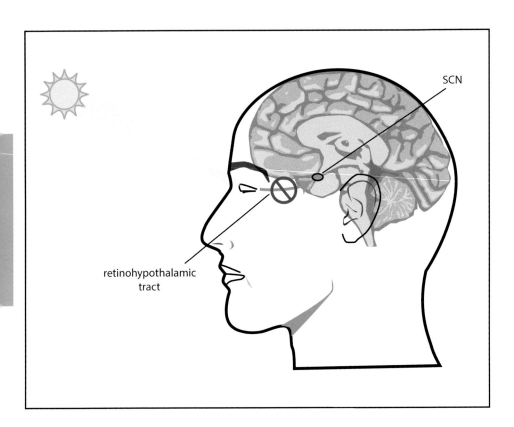

FIGURE 2.27. Non-24-Hour Sleep-Wake disorder is a circadian rhythm disorder that primarily affects individuals who are blind (Bonacci et al., 2015). Those who are visually impaired lack the ability to entrain the internal circadian clock with light acting on the suprachiasmatic nucleus (SCN) via the retinohypothalamic tract (RHT). This free-running internal clock leads to irregular sleep/wake patterns that may cause both insomnia and excessive daytime sleepiness. Recently, the melatonin MT1 and MT2 receptor agonist tasimelteon has been approved for the treatment of Non-24-Hour Sleep-Wake disorder. The actions of tasimelteon at MT2 receptors are thought to underlie its effectiveness at retraining the circadian clock (Bonacci et al., 2015; Carocci et al., 2014; Laudon and Frydman-Marom, 2014).

Obstructive Sleep Apnea

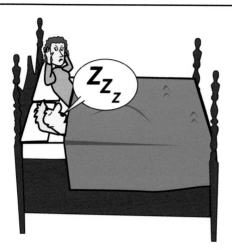

Clinical Features

- Loud snoring
- Obesity
- Hypertension
- Neck >17"
- Enlarged tonsils
- Loss of interest
- Excessive daytime sleepiness
- Fatigue
- Depression

Pathophysiology

- Partial/full collapse of upper airway
- Narrowing may occur at different levels
- Muscle tone, airway reflexes
- Metabolic abnormalities in frontal lobe white matter and hippocampus

FIGURE 2.28. Approximately 1 out of 15 adults suffer with moderate obstructive sleep apnea (OSA), and as many as 75% of individuals with insomnia have a sleep-related breathing disorder. Having OSA can nearly double general medical expenses, mainly due to the association of OSA with cardiovascular disease. Features of OSA include episodes of complete (apnea) or partial (hypopnea) upper airway obstruction that result in decreased blood oxygen saturation; these episodes are terminated by arousal (Abad and Guilleminault, 2011; Black et al., 2010; Krakow and Ulibarri, 2012; Tarasiuk and Reuveni, 2013; O'Donoghue et al., 2012; Lim and Veasey, 2010; Norman et al., 2012).

Diagnosing Obstructive Sleep Apnea

APNEA-HYPOPNEA INDEX (AHI)

$$AHI = \frac{(hypopneas + apneas) \times 60}{Total\ sleep\ time\ (minutes)}$$

RESPIRATORY DISTURBANCE INDEX (RDI)

$$RDI = \frac{(Respiratory\ effort\text{-}related\ arousals + hypopneas + apneas) \times 60}{Total\ sleep\ time\ (minutes)}$$

AHI or RDI 5-15 = mild sleep apnea
AHI or RDI 15-30 = moderate sleep apnea
AHI or RDI >30 = severe sleep apnea

FIGURE 2.29. The diagnosis of obstructive sleep apnea may involve the use of polysomnography (PSG), and recent advancements in technology allow for in-home use of a portable monitor; this option is more cost effective but perhaps less accurate. The frequency of obstructive events is measured with either the Apnea-Hypopnea Index (AHI) or the Respiratory Disturbance Index (RDI). Unlike the AHI, the RDI takes into account respiratory events that disrupt sleep but are not technically hypopneas or apneas (respiratory effort-related arousals, or RERAs). The Multiple Sleep Latency Test (MSLT) is not routinely indicated unless symptoms persist despite treatment (Ahmed et al., 2007; Epstein et al., 2009).

Restless Legs Syndrome

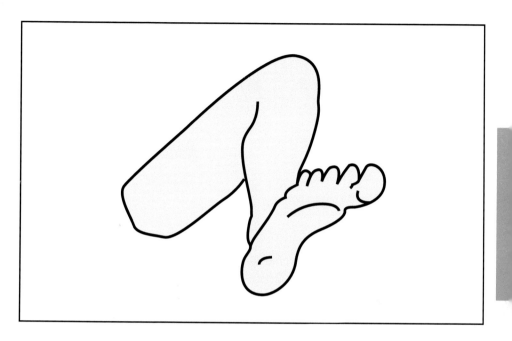

FIGURE 2.30. Restless legs syndrome (RLS) affects 2-3% of the population and is twice as common in women. The symptoms of RLS include an urge to move the lower limbs (associated with paresthesias or dysesthesias) and typically worsen during periods of rest. In addition to the physical discomfort of RLS, patients often experience both excessive daytime sleepiness and insomnia (specifically, impaired sleep onset and maintenance) that interfere with daily functioning. Deficiencies in dopamine and iron have both been associated with RLS; thus, various treatment options target the dopaminergic system, and iron supplementation may be effective. Periodic limb movements (PLMs) are also involuntary muscle activations that occur at intervals of 5-90 seconds and last 0.5-15 seconds. Nearly 90% of individuals with RLS also have PLMs; however, most individuals with PLMs do not have RLS. Although the etiology and neurobiology of PLMs may differ from those of RLS, treatment strategies are similar for the 2 disorders (Burke and Faulkner, 2011; Freedom, 2011; Stahl, 2013).

Neurobiology of Restless Legs Syndrome

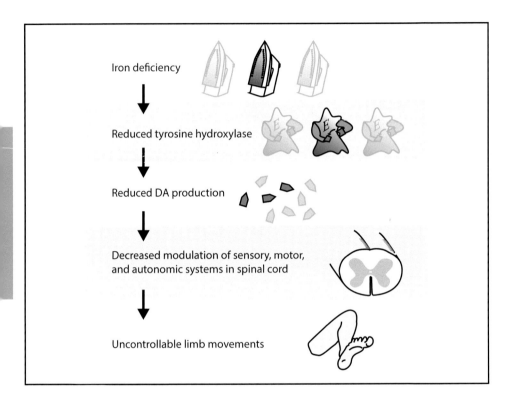

Iron deficiency

Reduced tyrosine hydroxylase

Reduced DA production

Decreased modulation of sensory, motor, and autonomic systems in spinal cord

Uncontrollable limb movements

FIGURE 2.31. Although the full etiology of restless legs syndrome (RLS) has yet to be elucidated, primary RLS appears to be familial, whereas secondary RLS is commonly seen with iron deficiency, renal failure, pregnancy, and multiple sclerosis; however, even in non-familial cases, a strong heritability is evidenced. Iron deficiency in particular shares a strong relationship with RLS; it is hypothesized that reduced levels of iron—a critical cofactor for tyrosine hydroxylase, the enzyme responsible for dopamine production—leads to lower dopamine (DA) production and release in the spinal cord. As discussed in Chapter 1, DA fluctuates with a circadian rhythm, and DA levels are at their lowest in the evening. It has therefore been hypothesized that during the evening hours, when DA is at its nadir, dopaminergic neurotransmission is especially low, leading to reduced dopaminergic modulation of the sensory, motor, and autonomic systems in the spinal cord (Frenette, 2011; Miletic and Relja, 2011; Thorpe et al., 2011; Seghal and Mignot, 2011; Freedom, 2011).

Sample Questions from the Cambridge-Hopkins Diagnostic Questionnaire for RLS (CH-RLSq)

1. Do you have, or have you had, recurrent uncomfortable feelings or sensations in your legs while you are seated or lying down?
   - Yes • No

2. Do you, or have you had, a recurrent need or urge to move your legs while you were sitting or lying down?
   - Yes • No

3. Are you more likely to have these feelings when you are resting (either sitting or lying down) or when you are physically active?
   - Resting • Active

4. If you get up or move around when you have these feeling do these feelings get any better while you actually keep moving?
   - Yes • No • Don't know

5. Which times of day are these feelings in your legs most likely to occur (Please circle one or more than one)
   - Morning • Mid-day • Afternoon • Evening • Night • About equal at all times

6. Will simply changing leg position by itself once without continuing to move usually relieve these feelings?
   - Usually relieves • Does not usually relieve

7a. Are these feelings ever due to muscle cramps?
   - Yes • No • Don't know

7b. If so, are they always due to muscle cramps?
   - Yes • No • Don't know

Scoring: Definite RLS: 1 yes, 2 yes, 3 resting, 4 yes, 5 NOT equal or morning, 6 does not usually relieve, 7a as no OR 7b as no

FIGURE 2.32. When diagnosing restless legs syndrome, the Cambridge-Hopkins Diagnostic Questionnaire for RLS (CH-RLSq) is useful (Allen et al., 2009). Additionally, thyroid and liver functioning as well as levels of folate, vitamin B12, and blood sugar should be measured. Immobilization testing, in which leg activity and an electroencephalogram (EEG) are recorded before bedtime; polysomnography; and actigraphy are often useful for determining the existence and severity of RLS (Miletic and Relja, 2011; Gupta et al., 2014).

Treatment of Sleep/Wake Disorders

In Chapter 3, we discuss numerous pharmacological and nonpharmacological strategies for treating sleep/wake disturbances. We address methods for resetting circadian rhythms that are out of sync with environmental cues, treatments for disorders of both hypersomnia and insomnia, and strategies for addressing obstructive sleep apnea and restless legs syndrome. It is important to stress that sleep/wake disorders often coexist within the same individual, and a multimodal treatment approach may be the best way to optimize outcomes for the individual patient.

Resetting Circadian Rhythms

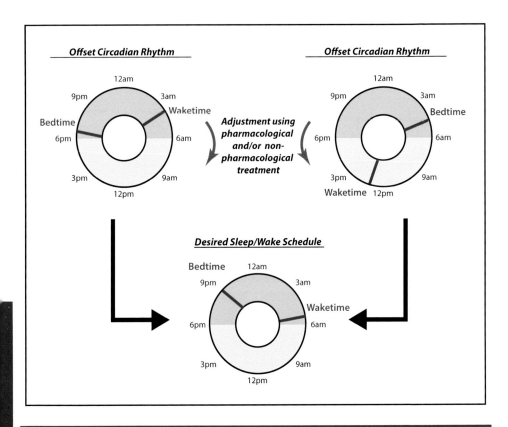

FIGURE 3.1. There are several pharmacological and nonpharmacological strategies that may be effective for synchronizing the internal clock with external environmental and social cues. These strategies may be useful in the treatment of circadian rhythm disorders, such as advanced or delayed sleep phase disorder (ASPD and DSPD), Non-24-Hour Sleep-Wake disorder, and shift work disorder; many may also be beneficial in ameliorating the symptoms of insomnia and hypersomnia (Mokhlesi and Gozal, 2011; Liira et al., 2014; Tahara and Shibata, 2014).

Sleep Hygiene

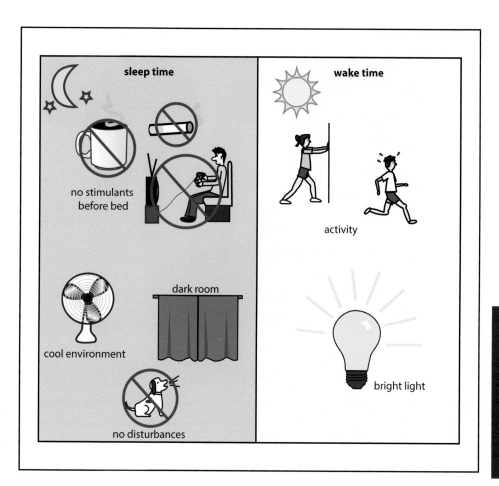

FIGURE 3.2. Good sleep hygiene involves using the bed exclusively for sleep as opposed to activities such as reading or watching television; avoiding stimulants such as alcohol, caffeine, and nicotine as well as strenuous exercise before bed; limiting time spent awake in bed (if not asleep within 20 minutes, one should get up and return to bed when sleepy); not watching the clock; adopting regular sleep habits; and avoiding light at night (Stahl, 2013). In the case of narcolepsy, scheduled naps of 15–20 minutes may also be beneficial (Harris et al., 2012).

Melatonergic Agents

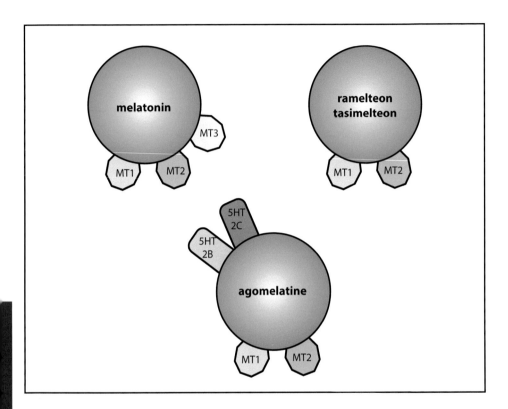

FIGURE 3.3. As discussed in Chapter 1, melatonin acts as a zeitgeber to reset circadian rhythms. When given at the appropriate time, melatonin (or a melatonin agonist) may help promote sleep by resetting the sleep/wake cycle. There are several different chronobiotic agents that act at melatonin receptors, as shown here. Melatonin itself, available over the counter, acts at MT1 and MT2 receptors as well as at the melatonin 3 (MT3) site. Both ramelteon and tasimelteon are MT1 and MT2 receptor agonists and seem to improve sleep onset, though not necessarily sleep maintenance. Agomelatine is not only an MT1 and MT2 receptor agonist, but also a 5HT2C and 5HT2B receptor antagonist; it is available as an antidepressant in Europe (Stahl, 2013). Ramelteon was recently approved by the FDA for the treatment of insomnia, and tasimelteon was recently FDA-approved for the treatment of Non-24-Hour Sleep-Wake disorder (Stahl, 2013; Bonacci et al., 2015).

Bright Light Therapy

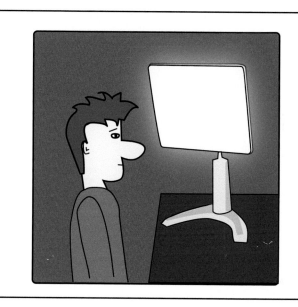

FIGURE 3.4. As discussed in Chapter 1, exposure to light alters circadian rhythms and suppresses melatonin release. It is therefore not surprising that treatment with 10,000 lux, bright, blue light for 30 minutes a day may be used to reset circadian rhythms. Importantly, the administration of bright light therapy must be appropriately timed in accordance with the patient's circadian phase of melatonin secretion, with light administration occurring approximately 8 hours after evening melatonin secretion or in accordance with a predetermined bright light phase response curve (Khalsa et al., 2003). One form of bright light therapy, dawn simulation therapy, applies a slow, incremental light signal at the end of the sleep cycle (Dallaspezia and Benedetti, 2011; Pail et al., 2011). Data show that performance, alertness, and mood during the night shift can be improved in shift workers using bright light re-entrainment of circadian rhythms (Crowley et al., 2004).

Promoting Sleep

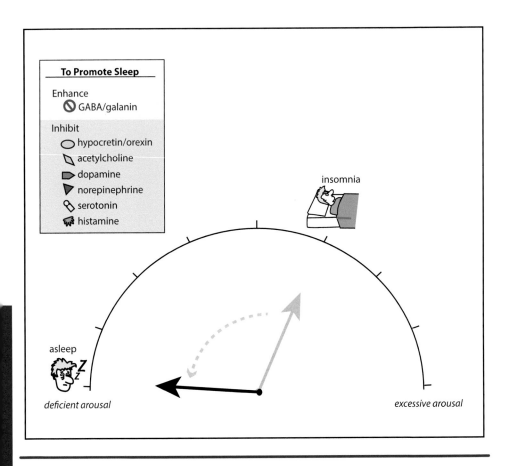

FIGURE 3.5. Agents that reduce brain activation, such as positive allosteric modulators of GABA-A receptors (e.g., benzodiazepines, "Z-drugs"), histamine 1 antagonists, and serotonin 2A/2C antagonists, can shift one's arousal state from hyperactive to asleep (Espana and Scammell, 2011).

Nonpharmacological Treatments for Insomnia

RELAXATION TRAINING
Aimed to reduce somatic tension and intrusive thoughts that interfere with sleep

STIMULUS CONTROL THERAPY
Get out of bed if not sleepy; use bed only for sleeping; no napping

SLEEP RESTRICTION THERAPY
Limit time spent in bed to produce mild sleep deprivation; results in more consolidated sleep

INTENSIVE SLEEP RETRAINING
25-hour sleep deprivation period in which the patient is given 50 sleep onset trials but awoken following 3 minutes of sleep

COGNITIVE BEHAVIORAL THERAPY
Reduce negative attitudes and misconceptions about sleep

FIGURE 3.6. There are several nonpharmacological treatment options for patients with insomnia. Among these are relaxation training, stimulus control therapy, sleep restriction therapy, intensive sleep retraining, and cognitive behavioral therapy (CBT) for insomnia (Harris et al., 2012; Morin and Benca, 2012). Cognitive behavioral therapy for insomnia has been shown to have beneficial effects on several sleep parameters, including sleep efficiency and sleep quality, as well as depression (Koffel et al., 2014).

Pharmacological Treatments for Insomnia

Pharmacological Agent	FDA-Approved for Insomnia
Benzodiazepine Hypnotics	
Estazolam	√
Flurazepam	√
Quazepam	√
Temazepam	√
Triazolam	√
Nonbenzodiazepine Hypnotics	
Eszopiclone	√
Zaleplon	√
Zolpidem	√
Antidepressants	
Doxepin	√
Trazodone	
Hypocretin/Orexin Antagonist	
Suvorexant	√
Melatonin Receptor Agonists	
Melatonin	
Ramelteon	√
Tasimelteon	
Antipsychotics	
Quetiapine	
Olanzapine	
Anticonvulsants	
Clonazepam	
Gabapentin	
Tiagabine	

FIGURE 3.7. Pharmacological agents used in the treatment of insomnia include benzodiazepine and nonbenzodiazepine hypnotics as well as an orexin antagonist, antidepressants, antipsychotics, and anticonvulsants. In many cases, a combination of agents may be required to optimize symptom control in patients with insomnia (Richey and Krystal, 2011).

Benzodiazepine Hypnotics

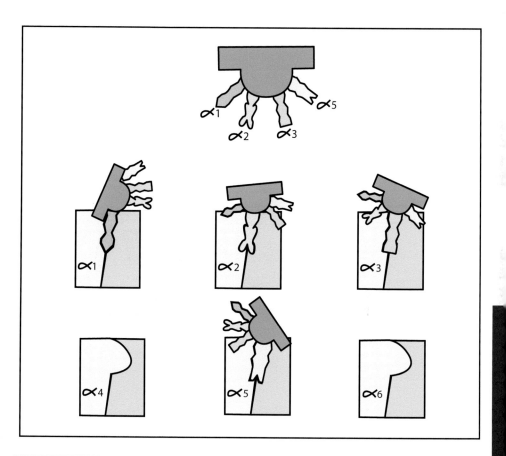

FIGURE 3.8. The benzodiazepine hypnotics all bind to α1, α2, α3, and α5 subunits of the GABA-A receptor. However, α subunit expression differs throughout the brain, and it is the selectivity for various α subunits that lends individual benzodiazepines their assorted effects outside of sedation (e.g., anxiolytic, anti-pain) (Gravielle, 2015). All benzodiazepines carry a high risk of tolerance and withdrawal effects and are therefore not recommended for the long-term treatment of insomnia (Stahl, 2013).

Nonbenzodiazepine Hypnotics

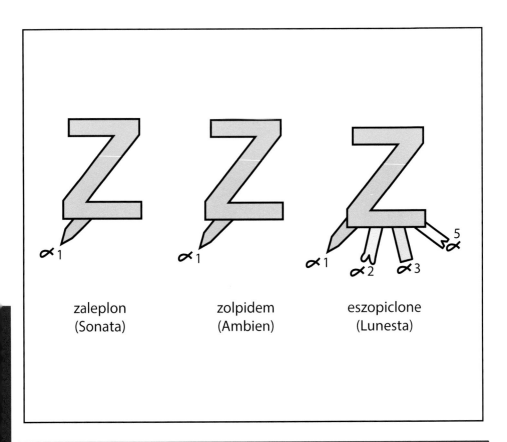

zaleplon
(Sonata)

zolpidem
(Ambien)

eszopiclone
(Lunesta)

FIGURE 3.9. Unlike the benzodiazepine hypnotics, the nonbenzodiazepine hypnotics (also known as "Z-drugs"), including zaleplon and zolpidem, bind selectively to 1 or 2 α subunits of the GABA-A receptor. The selectivity of nonbenzodiazepines is hypothesized to underlie the non-sedative properties of individual agents. For example, binding to α2 and α3 subunits may impart anxiolytic, antidepressant, and anti-pain effects. Another Z-drug, eszopiclone, does not bind selectively; however, the binding of eszopiclone is different from that of benzodiazepine hypnotics. Therefore, Z-drugs are believed to carry less risk of tolerance than benzodiazepine hypnotics; in fact, eszopiclone is the only hypnotic agent approved for use over 35 days (Stahl, 2013).

Antidepressants

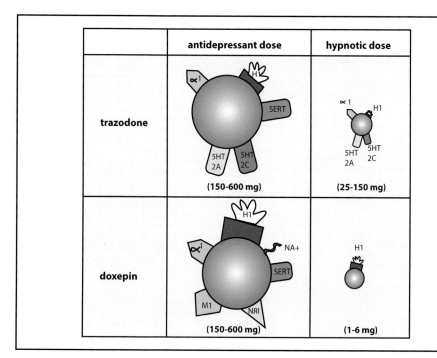

FIGURE 3.10. At antidepressant doses (150–600 mg/day), trazodone is a serotonin reuptake inhibitor and has serotonin 2A and 2C antagonism. In addition, trazodone is an antagonist at histamine 1 and alpha 1 adrenergic receptors, which can make it very sedating, particularly when given at antidepressant doses during the day. At low doses (25–150 mg/day), trazodone does not adequately block serotonin reuptake but retains its other properties; thus, it can still be sedating. However, because trazodone has a relatively short half-life (6–8 hours), if dosed only once daily at night, it can improve sleep without having daytime effects.

Doxepin is a tricyclic antidepressant (TCA) that at antidepressant doses (150–300 mg/day) inhibits serotonin and norepinephrine reuptake and is an antagonist at histamine 1, muscarinic 1, and alpha 1 adrenergic receptors. At low doses (1–6 mg/day), however, doxepin is quite selective for histamine 1 receptors and thus may be used as a hypnotic. Doxepin may improve sleep in the last hour of an 8-hour night without residual daytime impairment; however, it may exacerbate symptoms of restless legs syndrome (RLS) (Stahl, 2013).

Hypothetical Actions of Hypocretin/Orexin Antagonists

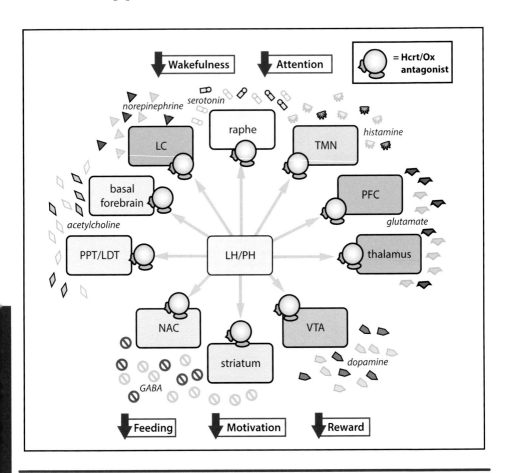

FIGURE 3.11. Hypocretin/orexins have excitatory actions on various brain areas, stimulating the release of an assortment of neurotransmitters involved in wakefulness and arousal as well as feeding, motivation, and reward behaviors. The blockade of hypocretin/orexin receptors via hypocretin/orexin antagonists may therefore not only be useful for the treatment of insomnia (by reducing wakefulness), but may also have therapeutic value for the treatment of disorders of addiction, compulsivity, and overeating/obesity (Scammel and Winrow, 2011).

Hypocretin/Orexin Antagonists

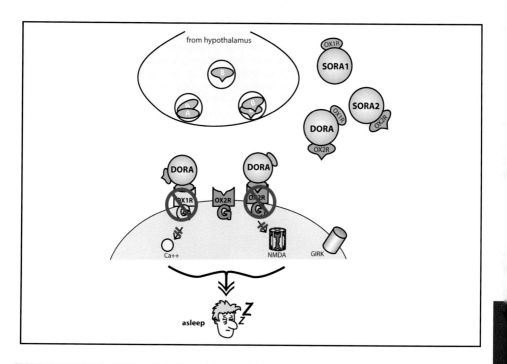

FIGURE 3.12. The stimulation of hypocretin/orexin receptors is hypothesized to sustain wakefulness and increase arousal in motivating conditions. Antagonism of the Hcrt-1 (OxR1) receptor is believed to modulate dopamine in addiction/reward centers of the brain, whereas antagonism of Hcrt-2 (OxR2) receptors may decrease histamine activity in the hypothalamus (Bonnavion and de Lecca, 2010; Brisbare-Roch et al., 2007; Espana and Scammell, 2011; Ruoff et al., 2011; Hoever et al., 2012; Equihua et al., 2013; Hoyer and Jacobson, 2013; Wei Yeoh et al., 2014). Given that hypocretin/orexin antagonists promote sleep without acting directly on GABA receptors, it is hypothesized that hypocretin/orexin antagonists will have fewer side effects than many earlier-generation hypnotics (Scammell and Winrow, 2011).

One dual hypocretin/orexin antagonist (DORA; blocking both Hcrt-1 and Hcrt-2 receptors), suvorexant, was recently approved for the treatment of insomnia following several trials showing efficacy in promoting sleep without causing rebound insomnia or risk of dependence (Herring et al., 2016; Dubey et al., 2015; Bennett et al., 2014; Michaelson et al., 2014).

Antipsychotics and Anticonvulsants

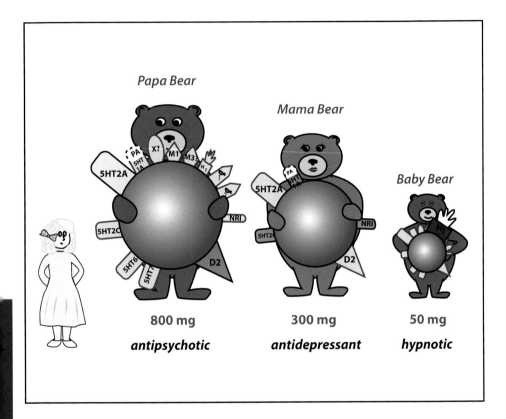

FIGURE 3.13. Although antipsychotics are not FDA-approved for promoting sleep, atypical antipsychotics (olanzapine and quetiapine in particular) are sometimes used "off label" for this purpose. The sedating properties of these antipsychotic agents are hypothesized to stem from their strong binding and antagonist properties at various receptors, including the histamine H1 receptor. Often, a low dose of, for instance, quetiapine can be used as a sedative without instigating the antipsychotic and side effect qualities attributed to dopamine D2 receptor antagonism (Stahl, 2013).

Anticonvulsants are also not FDA-approved for the treatment of insomnia but are often prescribed off label in order to promote sleep. The sedative properties of anticonvulsants such as clonazepam, gabapentin, and tiagabine are thought to arise from their effects on GABAergic neurotransmission (Dresler et al., 2014; Morin and Benca, 2012).

Promoting Wakefulness

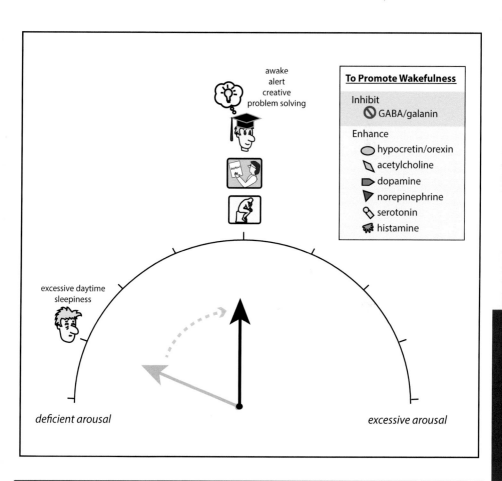

FIGURE 3.14. Agents that increase brain activation, such as the stimulants modafinil and caffeine, can shift one's arousal state from hypoactive to awake with normal alertness (Stahl, 2013). The currently available agents as well as those in development for the treatment of excessive sleepiness target the neurotransmitter systems involved in the sleep and wake circuits, inhibiting the neurotransmitters that promote sleep and/or enhancing the systems that promote wakefulness.

Pharmacological Treatments for Hypersomnia

	Excessive Daytime Sleepiness	Cataplexy
Stimulants		
Amphetamine	*√	
Methylphenidate	*√	
Lisdexamfetamine	√	
Atomoxetine	√	√
Antidepressants		
TCA - Protriptyline		√
TCA - Imipramine		√
TCA - Clomipramine		√
TCA - Desipramine		√
SNRI - Venlafaxine		√
SNRI - Duloxetine		√
SSRI - Fluoxetine		√
MAOI - Selegiline	√	√
Other Agents		
Modafinil/Armodafinil	*√	
Sodium Oxybate	*√	*√
Caffeine	√	
* Indicates FDA approval for this indication		

FIGURE 3.15. Pharmacological agents used in the treatment of excessive daytime sleepiness and cataplexy include stimulants and antidepressants as well as sodium oxybate and the wake-promoting agent modafinil/armodafinil (Hirai and Nishino, 2011; Mignot, 2012; Thorpy and Dauvilliers, 2014; Zaharna et al., 2010). In many cases, a combination of agents may be required to optimize symptom control in patients with hypersomnia.

Stimulants

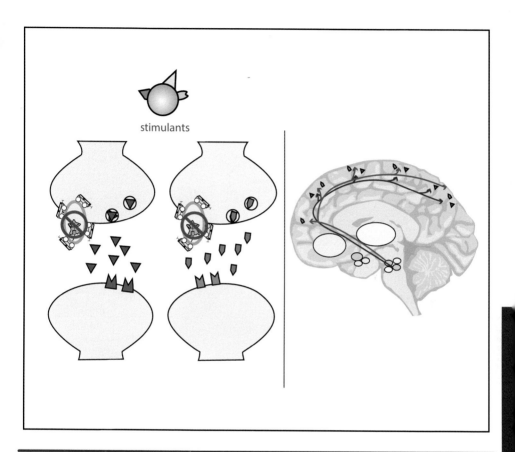

FIGURE 3.16. Stimulants, including amphetamine and methylphenidate, act in part by inhibiting dopamine (DA) and/or norepinephrine (NE) reuptake transporters (DAT and NET, respectively), thus increasing the levels of DA and NE in the wake circuit. Atomoxetine has a similar mechanism of action involving the inhibition of NE reuptake (Hirai and Nishino, 2011; Mignot, 2012).

Antidepressants

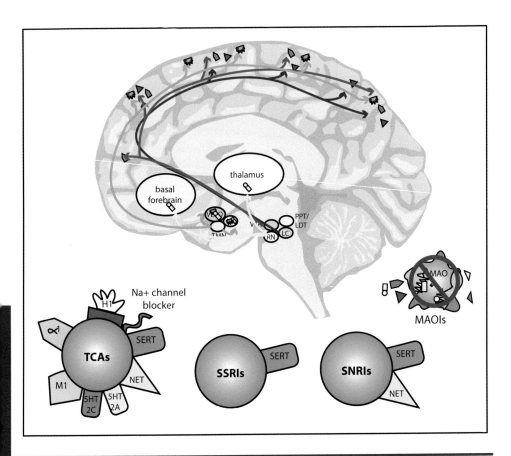

FIGURE 3.17. Antidepressants, including tricyclic antidepressants (TCAs), selective serotonin reuptake inhibitors (SSRIs), and serotonin-norepinephrine reuptake inhibitors (SNRIs), can have beneficial effects on cataplexy by reducing REM sleep. Although monoamine oxidase inhibitors (MAOIs) are perhaps underutilized, there is some evidence to suggest that selegiline may have efficacy in the treatment of both excessive sleepiness and cataplexy (Ahmed and Thorpy, 2010). In addition to its antidepressant actions, selegiline may be useful in treating cataplexy because it is metabolized into the stimulant amphetamine. However, it is important to note that the cessation of antidepressant treatment may result in rebound cataplexy (Mignot, 2012).

Modafinil/Armodafinil

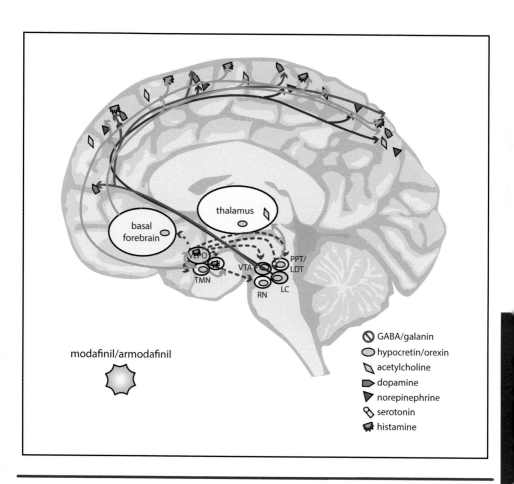

FIGURE 3.18. Although the exact mechanisms by which modafinil and its R-enantiomer, armodafinil, decrease sleepiness are not fully understood, evidence suggests that these agents promote wakefulness by acting directly or indirectly on many components of the sleep/wake circuit. Modafinil and armodafinil are hypothesized to inhibit GABA and promote dopamine, norepinephrine, histamine, and hypocretin/orexin (Morrissette, 2013; Bogan, 2010; Darwish et al., 2010; Erman et al., 2011).

Modafinil/Armodafinil

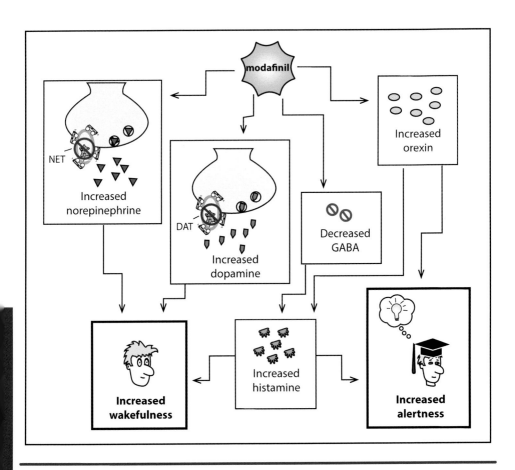

FIGURE 3.19. Modafinil and its R-enantiomer, armodafinil, increase both norepinephrine (NE) and dopamine (DA), possibly via their blockade of both the NE and DA reuptake transporters (NET and DAT, respectively). The actions of NE at alpha-adrenergic receptors and DA at dopamine D2 receptors are thought to contribute to the wake-promoting properties of modafinil. Orexin is a key component of the arousal system; thus, the hypothesized action of modafinil on the orexinergic system may help increase alertness. Additionally, modafinil may indirectly increase histamine, either by reducing GABAergic inhibition of histaminergic neurons or via actions at orexinergic neurons. The increase in histamine may contribute to both the wake-promoting effects of modafinil as well as the potential of modafinil to increase alertness (Morrissette, 2013; Darwish et al., 2012; He et al., 2011).

Sodium Oxybate

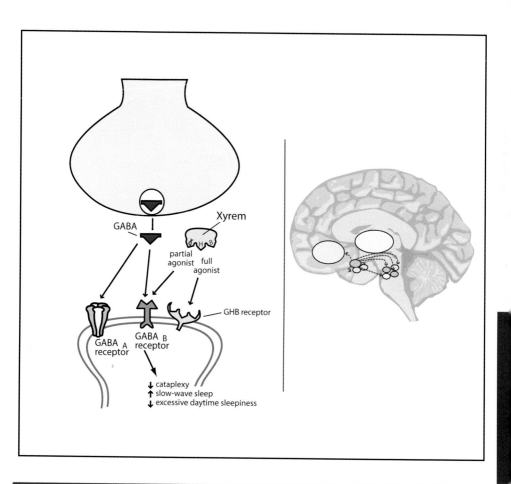

FIGURE 3.20. Sodium oxybate, also known as gamma-hydroxybutyrate (GHB), is a full agonist at gamma-hydroxybutyrate receptors and a partial agonist at GABA-B receptors. As a GABA-B partial agonist, sodium oxybate acts as an antagonist when GABA levels are elevated and as an agonist when GABA levels are low. It is hypothesized that sodium oxybate increases slow-wave sleep and improves cataplexy via these actions at GABA-B receptors. Sodium oxybate is approved for use in both cataplexy and excessive sleepiness, and it appears to enhance slow-wave sleep and reduce hypnagogic hallucinations and sleep paralysis (Stahl, 2013; Hirai and Nishino, 2011; Adenuga and Attarian, 2014).

Caffeine

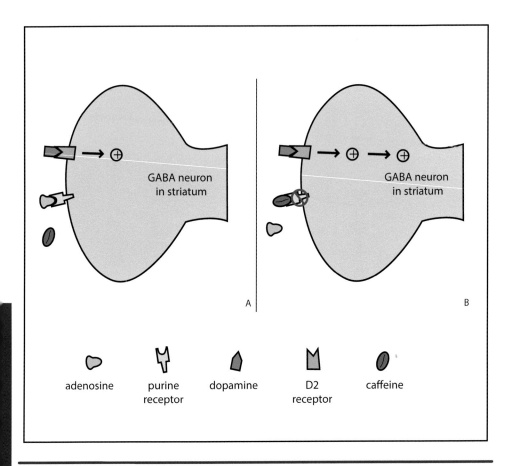

FIGURE 3.21. A) Both adenosine 2A receptors and dopamine D2 receptors are localized on GABAergic neurons in the striatum, forming a heteromeric complex. When adenosine stimulates adenosine 2A receptors, this reduces the affinity of nearby D2 receptors for dopamine. **B)** By blocking adenosine from binding to adenosine 2A receptors, caffeine prevents the lowered affinity of D2 receptors for dopamine. The increased GABAergic neurotransmission disinhibits downstream excitatory glutamatergic neurotransmission (Morrissette, 2013).

Emerging Treatments for Hypersomnia

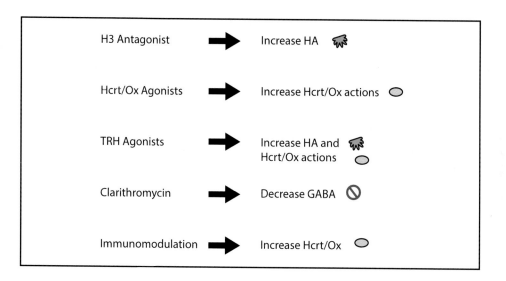

FIGURE 3.22. There are several agents currently being investigated for the treatment of hypersomnia (Cao, 2011). These include histamine H3 receptor antagonists, hypocretin/orexin (Hcrt/Ox) agonists, thyrotropin-releasing hormone (TRH) agonists, and the antibiotic clarithromycin. Additional treatment strategies include immunomodulation with immunoglobulins and the blockade of T-cell entry into the brain. Antagonism of the histamine H3 receptor may increase histamine neurotransmission, leading to enhancement of the wake circuit (Stahl, 2013; Broderick and Masri, 2011). Treatment with Hcrt/Ox agonists may be especially beneficial to patients with narcolepsy due to loss of Hcrt/Ox neurons; however, the development of an Hcrt/Ox agonist that readily crosses the blood-brain barrier has been unsuccessful so far (Adenuga and Attarian, 2014; Dauvilliers and Tafti, 2006; Hirai and Nishino, 2011; Mignot, 2012). Thyrotropin-releasing hormone (TRH) promotes histamine release from the tuberomammillary nucleus (TMN) and modulates Hcrt/Ox from the lateral hypothalamus (LH); therefore, TRH agonists may be effective in stimulating the wake circuitry on multiple levels (Gonzalez et al., 2009; Parmentier et al., 2009). Clarithromycin is an antibiotic that acts as a GABA-A receptor antagonist and may therefore reduce activation of the sleep circuit to promote wakefulness (Trotti et al., 2013; Trotti et al., 2015). Immunomodulation-based treatments seek to prevent the hypothesized autoimmune reaction that leads to the death of Hcrt/Ox (Dauvilliers et al., 2009; Knudsen et al., 2012; Griebel et al., 2012).

Treating Obstructive Sleep Apnea

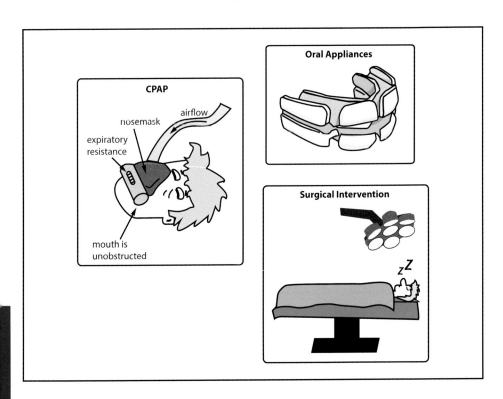

FIGURE 3.23. There are several treatment options available for managing obstructive sleep apnea (OSA). The first-line treatment option for OSA is continuous positive airway pressure (CPAP). Although CPAP treatment is quite effective and has been shown to reduce hospitalization rates and healthcare costs, adherence rates are poor (54%). For patients who find CPAP intolerable, there are other treatment options that may be considered, including bilevel positive airway pressure (BPAP), auto-titrating positive airway pressure (APAP), oral appliances designed to stabilize the jaw and/or tongue during sleep, and various surgeries aimed at correcting physical attributes that may contribute to OSA. Additionally, several behavioral interventions may be useful for ameliorating OSA; these include weight loss (BMI <25), exercise, the avoidance of alcohol and sedatives at bedtime, and positional therapy (i.e., the use of a backpack or other object that prevents the patient from sleeping on their back) (Epstein et al., 2009; Norman et al., 2012; Tarasiuk and Reuveni, 2013; Rogers, 2012; Aurora et al., 2012).

Treating Restless Legs Syndrome/ Periodic Limb Movements

RLS Treatment	FDA-Approve
Dopamine Agonists	
Ropinirole	√
Pramipexole	√
Carbidopa-levodopa	
Iron supplementation	
GABAergic Agents	
Gabapentin enacarbil	√
Pregabalin	
Opiates	
Benzodiazepines	

FIGURE 3.24. Treatment options for restless legs syndrome and periodic limb movements include dopamine agonists such as ropinirole, pramipexole, and carbidopa-levodopa. However, it is important to note that dopamine agonists may also increase the risk of impulsive behaviors and lead to worsening of symptoms. Iron supplementation may also be a useful treatment strategy, as RLS is hypothesized to stem from iron deficiency in some cases. GABAergic agents such as gabapentin/ pregabalin may also bring relief from symptoms of RLS; in fact, gabapentin enacarbil has recently been FDA-approved with once-daily dosing for the treatment of RLS. Additionally, low potency opiates and benzodiazepines are sometime used. Keep in mind that some medications, including antipsychotics, antiemetics, SSRIs, TCAs, lithium, antihistamines, calcium antagonists, and antihypertensives, may actually exacerbate symptoms of RLS (Freedom, 2011; Frenette, 2011; Miletic and Relja, 2011; Thorpe et al., 2011; Burke and Faulkner, 2011; Garcia-Borreguero et al., 2010; Oertel et al., 2011).

Stahl's Illustrated | Summary

As our understanding of the neurobiological and molecular bases of sleep expands, it is becoming increasingly clear that both the quality and quantity of sleep can greatly affect our physical and mental health; it is therefore critical that issues affecting sleep and wake be adequately recognized and appropriately managed. As the state of the science of sleep improves, so does our ability to differentially diagnose and effectively treat sleep/wake disorders. There are numerous pharmacological and nonpharmacological treatment options available that target various components of the sleep/wake circuit to improve sleep/wake issues. There are also several agents under investigation for their potential as treatments and possibly disease-modifying drugs for an assortment of sleep/wake disorders.

Abad VC, Guilleminault C. Pharmacological treatment of obstructive sleep apnea. Curr Pharm Design 2011;17(15):1418-25.

Adenuga O, Attarian H. Treatment of disorders of hypersomnolence Curr Treatment Options Neurol 2014;16:302.

Ahmed I, Thorpy M. Clinical features, diagnosis and treatment of narcolepsy. Clin Chest Med 2010;31:371-81.

Allen RP, Burchell BJ, MacDonald B, et al. Validation of the self-completed Cambridge-Hopkins questionnaire (CH-RLSq) for ascertainment of restless legs syndrome (RLS) in a population survey. Sleep Med 2009;10(10):1079-100.

Arallanes-Licea E, Caldelas I, De Ita-Pérez D, et al. The circadian timing system: a recent addition in the physiological mechanisms underlying pathological and aging processes. Aging Dis 2014;5(6):406-18.

Artioli P, Lorenzi C, Priovano A, et al. How do genes exert their role? Period 3 gene variants and possible influences on mood disorder phenotypes. Eur Neuropsychopharmacol 2007;17(9):587-94.

Aurora RN, Chowdhuri S, Ramar K, et al. The treatment of central sleep apnea syndromes in adults: practice parameters with an evidence-based literature review and meta-analyses. Sleep 2012;35(1):17-40.

Banerjee S, Wang Y, Solt LA, et al. Pharmacological targeting of the mammalian clock regulates sleep architecture and emotional behaviour. Nat Commun 2014;5:5759.

Barger LK, Ogeil RP, Drake CL, et al. Validation of a questionnaire to screen for shift work disorder. Sleep 2012;35(12):1693-703.

Bastien CH, Vallieres A, Morin CM. Validation of the Insomnia Severity Index as an outcome measure for insomnia research. Sleep Med 2001;2(4):297-307.

Benedetti F, Serretti A, Colombo C, et al. Influence of CLOCK gene polymorphisms on circadian mood fluctuation and illness recurrence in bipolar depression. Am J Med Genetics B Neuropsychiatr Genetics 2003;123B(1):23-6.

Bennett T, Bray D, Neville MW. Suvorexant, a dual orexin receptor antagonist for the management of insomnia. PT 2014;39(4):264-6.

Black JE, Hull SG, Tiller J, et al. The long-term tolerability and efficacy of armodafinil in patients with excessive sleepiness associated with treated obstructive sleep apnea, shift work disorder, or narcolepsy: an open-label extension study. J Clin Sleep Med 2010;6(5):458-66.

Bogan RK. Armodafinil in the treatment of excessive sleepiness. Expert Opinion Pharmacother 2010;11(6):993-1002.

Bonacci JM, Venci JV, Ghandi MA. Tasimelteon (HetliozTM): a new melatonin receptor agonist for the treatment of non-24 sleep-wake disorder. J Pharm Pract 2015;28(5):473-8.

Bonnavion P, de Lecea L. Hypocretins in the control of sleep and wakefulness. Curr Neurol Neurosci Rep 2010;10:174-9.

Bonnet MH, Burton GG, Arand DL. Physiological and medical findings in insomnia: implications for diagnosis and care. Sleep Med Rev 2014;18(1):95-8.

Bourgin P, Zeitzer JM, Mignot E. CSF hypocretin-1 assessment in sleep and neurological disorders. Lancet Neurol 2008;7(7):649-62.

Brancaccio M, Enoki R, Mazuki CN, et al. Network-mediated encoding of circadian time: the suprachiasmatic nucleus (SCN) from genes to neurons to circuits, and back. J Neurosci 2014;34(46):15192-9.

Brisbare-Roch C, Dingemanse J, Koberstein R, et al. Promotion of sleep by targeting the orexin system in rats, dogs and humans. Nat Med 2007;13(2):150-5.

Broderick M, Masri T. Histamine H3 receptor (H3R) antagonists and inverse agonists in the treatment of sleep disorders. Curr Pharm Design 2011;17:1426-9.

Burke RA, Faulkner MA. Gabapentin enacarbil for the treatment of restless legs syndrome (RLS). Expert Opinion Pharmacother 2011;12(18):2905-14.

Buysse DJ, Reynolds CF III, Monk TH, et al. The Pittsburgh Sleep Quality Index: a new instrument for psychiatric practice and research. Psychiatry Res 1989;28(2):193-213.

Cappuccio FP, D'Elia L, Strazzullo P, et al. Sleep duration and all-cause mortality: a systematic review and meta-analysis of prospective studies. Sleep 2010;33(5):585-92.

Carocci A, Catalano A, Sinicropi MS. Melatonergic drugs in development. Clin Pharmacol Adv Applications 2014;6:127-37.

Cermakian N, Lange T, Golombek D, et al. Crosstalk between the circadian clock circuitry and the immune system. Chronobiol Int 2013;30(7):870-88.

Cirelli C. The genetic and molecular regulation of sleep: from fruit flies to humans. Nat Rev Neurosci 2009;10(8):549-60.

Colwell CS. Linking neural activity and molecular oscillators in the SCN. Nat Rev Neurosci 2011;12(10):553-69.

Crowley SJ, Lee C, Tseng CY, et al. Complete or partial circadian re-entrainment improves performance, alertness, and mood during night-shift work. Sleep 2004;27(6):1077-87.

Dallaspezia S, Benedetti F. Chronobiological therapy for mood disorders. Expert Rev Neurother 2011;11(7):961-70.

Darwish M, Bond M, Ezzet F. Armodafinil in patients with excessive sleepiness associated with shift work disorder: a pharmacokinetic/pharmacodynamic model for predicting and comparing their concentration-effect relationships. J Clin Pharmacol 2012;52(9):1328-42.

Darwish M, Kirby M, D'Andrea DM, et al. Pharmacokinetics of armodafinil and modafinil after single and multiple doses in patients with excessive sleepiness associated with treated obstructive sleep apnea: a randomized, open-label, crossover study. Clin Ther 2010;32(12):2074-87.

Dauvilliers Y, Abril B, Mas E, et al. Normalization of hypocretin-1 in narcolepsy after intravenous immunoglobulin treatment. Neurology 2009;73(16):1333-4.

Dauvilliers Y, Tafti M. Molecular genetics and treatment of narcolepsy. Ann Med 2006;38:252-62.

De la Herrán-Arita, Garcia-Garcia F. Narcolepsy as an immune-mediated disease. Sleep Disord 2014;2014:792687.

de Lecea L, Huerta R. Hypocretin (orexin) regulation of sleep-to-wake transitions. Frontiers Pharmacol 2015;5(16):1-7.

Dresler M, Spoormaker VI, Beitinger P, et al. Neuroscience-driven discovery and development of sleep therapeutics. Pharmacol Ther 2014;141:300-34.

Dubey AK, Handu SS, Mediratta PK. Suvorexant: the first orexin receptor antagonist to treat insomnia. J Pharmacol Pharmacother 2015;6(2):118-21.

Eckel-Mahan KL, Patel VR, de Mateo S, et al. Reprogramming of the circadian clock by nutritional challenge. Cell 2013;155(7):1464-78.

Epstein LJ, Kristo D, Strollo PJ, et al. Clinical guideline for the evaluation, management and long-term care of obstructive sleep apnea in adults. J Clin Sleep Med 2009;5(3):263-76.

Equihua AC, De la Herrán-Arita AK, Drucker-Colin R. Orexin receptor antagonists as therapeutic agents for insomnia. Frontiers Pharmacol 2013;4(163):1-10.

Erman MK, Seiden DJ, Yang R, et al. Efficacy and tolerability of armodafinil: effect on clinical condition late in the shift and overall functioning of patients with excessive sleepiness associated with shift work disorder. JOEM 2011;53(12):1460-5.

España RA, Scammell TE. Sleep neurobiology from a clinical perspective. Sleep 2011;34(7):845-58.

Freedom T. Sleep-related movement disorders. Dis Month 2011;57:438-47.

Frenette E. Restless legs syndrome in children: a review and update on pharmacological options. Curr Pharm Design 2011;17:1436-42.

Froy O. Metabolism and circadian rhythms—implications for obesity. Endocr Rev 2010;31(1):1-24.

Garcia-Borreguero D, Allen R, Kohnen R, et al. Loss of response during long-term treatment of restless legs syndrome: guidelines approved by the International Restless Legs Syndrome Study Group for use in clinical trials. Sleep Med 2010;11:956-9.

Gravielle MC. Activation-induced regulation of GABAA receptors: is there a link with the molecular basis of benzodiazepine tolerance? Pharmacol Res 2015; Epub ahead of print.

Green CB, Takahashi JS, Bass J. The meter of metabolism. Cell 2008;134(5):728-42.

Griebel G, Decobert M, Jacquet A, et al. Awakening properties of newly discovered highly selective H3 receptor antagonists in rats. Behav Brain Res 2012;232(2):416-20.

Golombek DA, Casiraghi LP, Agostino PV, et al. The times they are a-changing: effects of circadian desynchronization on physiology and disease. J Physiol Paris 2013;107:310-22.

Gonzalez JA, Horjales-Araujo E, Fugger L, et al. Stimulation of orexin/ hypocretin neurons by thyrotropin-releasing hormone. J Physiol 2009;587(pt 6):1179-86.

Guo X, Zheng L, Wang J, et al. Epidemiological evidence for the link between sleep duration and high blood pressure: a systematic review and meta-analysis. Sleep Med 2013;14:324-32.

Gupta R, Zalai D, Spence DW, et al. When insomnia is not just insomnia: the deeper correlates of disturbed sleep with reference to DSM-5. Asian J Psychiatry 2014;12:23-30.

Hampp G, Ripperger JA, Houben T, et al. Regulation of monoamine oxidase A by circadian-clock components implies influence on mood. Curr Biol 2008;18(9):678-83.

Harris J, Lack L, Kemo K, et al. A randomized controlled trial of intensive sleep retraining (ISR): a brief conditioning treatment for chronic insomnia. Sleep 2012;35(1):49-60.

Harrison EM, Gorman MR. Changing the waveform of circadian rhythms: considerations for shift-work. 2012;3(72):1-7.

He B, Peng H, Zhao Y, et al. Modafinil treatment prevents REM sleep deprivation-induced brain function impairment by increasing MMP-9 expression. Brain Res 2011;1426:38-42.

Herring WJ, Connor KM, Ivgy-May N, et al. Suvorexant in patients with insomnia: results from two 3-month randomized controlled clinical trials. Biol Psychiatry 2016;79(2):136-48.

Hirai N, Nishino S. Recent advances in the treatment of narcolepsy. Curr Treatment Options Neurol 2011;13:437-57.

Hoever P, Dorffner G, Benes H, et al. Orexin receptor antagonism, a new sleep-enabling paradigm: a proof-of-concept clinical trial. Clin Pharmacol Ther 2012;91(6):975-85.

Horne JA, Östberg O. A self-assessment questionnaire to determine morningness-eveningness in human circadian rhythms. Int J Chronobiol 1976;4:97-100.

Hoyer D, Jacobson LH. Orexin in sleep, addiction, and more: is the perfect insomnia drug at hand? Neuropeptides 2013;47:477-88.

Johansson C, Willeit M, Smedh C, et al. Circadian clock-related polymorphisms in seasonal affective disorder and their relevance to diurnal preference. Neuropsychopharmacology 2003;28(4):734-9.

Jones BE, Hassani OK. The role of Hcrt/Orx and MCH neurons in sleep-wake state regulation. Sleep 2013;36(12):1769-72.

Khalsa SB, Jewett ME, Cajochen C, et al. A phase response curve to single bright light pulses in human subjects. J Physiol 2003;549(pt 3):945-52.

Knudsen S, Biering-Sørensen B, Kornum BR, et al. Early IVIg treatment has no effect on post-H1N1 narcolepsy phenotype or hypocretin deficiency. Neurology 2012;79(1):102-3.

Koffel EA, Koffel JB, Gehrman PR. A meta-analysis of group cognitive behavioral therapy for insomnia. Sleep Med Rev 2015;19:6-16.

Krakow B, Ulibarri VA. Prevalence of sleep breathing complaints reported by treatment-seeking chronic insomnia disorder patients on presentation to a sleep medical center: a preliminary report. Sleep Breathing 2013;17(1):317-22.

Kripke DE, Nievergelt CM, Joo E, et al. Circadian polymorphisms associated with affective disorders. J Circadian Rhythms 2009;27:2.

Krystal AD, Benca RM, Kilduff TS. Understanding the sleep-wake cycle: sleep, insomnia, and the orexin system. J Clin Psychiatry 2013;74(suppl 1):3-20.

Krystal AD, Harsh JR, Yang R, et al. A double-blind, placebo-controlled study of armodafinil for excessive sleepiness in patients with treated obstructive sleep apnea and comorbid depression. J Clin Psychiatry 2010;71(1):32-40.

Lallukka T, Kaikkonen R., Härkänen T, et al. Sleep and sickness absence: a nationally representative register-based follow-up study. Sleep 2014;37(9):1413-25.

Larson-Prior LJ, Ju Y, Galvin JE. Cortical-subcortical interactions in hypersomnia disorders: mechanisms underlying cognitive and behavioral aspects of the sleep-wake cycle. Frontiers Neurol 2014;5(165):1-13.

Laudon M, Frydman-Marom A. Therapeutic effects of melatonin receptor agonists on sleep and comorbid disorders. Int J Mol Sci 2014;15:15924-50.

Liira J, Verbeek JH, Costa G, et al. Pharmacological interventions for sleepiness and sleep disturbances caused by shift work. Cochrane Database Syst Rev 2014;8:CD009776.

Lim DC, Veasey SC. Neural injury in sleep apnea. Curr Neurol Neurosci Rep 2010;10:47-52.

Liu Y, Wheaton AG, Chapman DP, et al. Sleep duration and chronic disease among US adults age 45 years and older: evidence from the 2010 behavioral risk factor surveillance system. Sleep 2013;36(10):1421-7.

Mahler SV, Moorman DE, Smith RJ, et al. Motivational activation: a unifying hypothesis of orexin/hypocretin function. Nat Neurosci 2014;17(10):1298-303.

Mansour HA, Wood J, Logue T, et al. Association of eight circadian genes with bipolar I disorder, schizoaffective disorder and schizophrenia. Genes Brain Behav 2006;5(2):150-7.

Martin JL, Hakim AD. Wrist actigraphy. Chest 2011;139(6):1514-27.

Masri S, Kinouchi K, Sassone-Corsi P. Circadian clocks, epigenetics, and cancer. Curr Opinion Oncology 2015;27:50-6.

Meyer JH, Ginovart N, Boovariwala A, et al. Elevated monoamine oxidase A levels in the brain: an explanation for the monoamine imbalance of major depression. Arch Gen Psychiatry 2006;63(11):1209-16.

Michelson D, Snyder E, Paradis E, et al. Safety and efficacy of suvorexant during 1-year treatment of insomnia with subsequent abrupt treatment discontinuation: a phase 3 randomised, double-blind, placebo-controlled trial. Lancet Neurol 2014;13:461-71.

Mignot EJM. A practical guide to the therapy of narcolepsy and hypersomnia syndromes. Neurotherapeutics 2012;9:739-52.

Miletic V, Relja M. Restless legs syndrome. Collegium Antropologicum 2011;35(4):1339-47.

Mokhlesi B, Gozal D. Update in sleep medicine 2010. Am J Respir Crit Care Med 2011;183:1472-6.

Morgenthaler TI, Kapur VK, Brown T, et al. Practice parameters for the treatment of narcolepsy and other hypersomnias of central origin. Sleep 2007;30(12):1705-11.

Morgenthaler TI, Lee-Chiong T, Alessi C, et al. Practice parameters for the clinical evaluation and treatment of circadian rhythm sleep disorders. Sleep 2007b;30(11):1445-59.

Morin CM, Benca R. Chronic insomnia. Lancet 2012;379:1129-41.

Morrissette DA. Twisting the night away: a review of the neurobiology, genetics, diagnosis, and treatment of shift work disorder. CNS Spectrums 2013;18(suppl 1):45-53.

Niervergelt CM, Kripke DF, Barrett TB, et al. Suggestive evidence for association of circadian genes PERIOD3 and ARNTL with bipolar disorder. Am J Med Genetics B Neuropsychiatr Genetics 2006;141B(3):234-41.

Nixon JP, Mavanji V, Butterick TA, et al. Sleep disorders, obesity, and aging: the role of orexin. Aging Res Rev 2015;20:63-73.

Norman D, Haberman PB, Valladares EM. Medical consequences and associations with untreated sleep-related breathing disorders and outcomes of treatments. J CA Dent Assoc 2012;40(2):141-9.

O'Donoghue FJ, Wellard RM, Rochford PD, et al. Magnetic resonance spectroscopy and neurocognitive dysfunction in obstructive sleep apnea before and after CPAP treatment. Sleep 2012;35(1):41-8.

Oertel W, Trenkwalder C, Benes H, et al. Long-term safety and efficacy of rotigotine transdermal patch for moderate-to-severe idiopathic restless legs syndrome: a 5-year open-label extension study. Lancet Neurol 2011;10:710-20.

Ohayon MM. Determining the level of sleepiness in the American population and its correlates. J Psychiatr Res 2012;46:422-7.

Oosterman JE, Kalsbeek A, la Fleur SE, et al. Impact of nutrition on circadian rhythmicity. Am J Physiol Regul Integrative Comp Physiol 2015;308(5):R337-50.

Orzel-Gryglewska J. Consequences of sleep deprivation. Int J Occup Med Environ Health 2010;23(1):95-114.

Pail G, Huf W, Pjrek E, et al. Bright-light therapy in the treatment of mood disorders. Neuropsychobiology 2011;64(3):152-62.

Palagini L, Biber K, Riemann D. The genetics of insomnia—evidence for epigenetic mechanisms? Sleep Med Rev 2014;18(3):225-35.

Palma JA, Urrestarazu E, Iriarte J. Sleep loss as a risk factor for neurologic disorders: a review. Sleep Med 2013;14:229-36.

Parmentier R, Kolbaev S, Klyuch BP, et al. Excitation of histaminergic tuberomammillary neurons by thyrotropin-releasing hormone. J Neurosci 2009;29(14):4471-83.

Parthasarathy S, Vasquez MM, Halonen M, et al. Persistent insomnia is associated with mortality risk. Am J Med 2015;128(3):268-75.

Partonen T, Treutlein J, Alpman A, et al. Three circadian clock genes Per2, Arntl, and Npas2 contribute to winter depression. Ann Med 2007;39(3):229-38.

Pigeon WR, Pinquart M, Conner K. Meta-analysis of sleep disturbance and suicidal thoughts and behaviors. J Clin Psychiatry 2012;73(9):e1160-7.

Pinto Jr LR, Alves RC, Caixeta E, et al. New guidelines for diagnosis and treatment of insomnia. Arq Neuropsiquiatr 2010;68(4):666-75.

Plante DT. Sleep propensity in psychiatric hypersomnolence: a systematic review and meta-analysis of multiple sleep latency findings. Sleep Med Rev 2016; Epub ahead of print.

Qureshi IA, Mehler MF. Epigenetics of sleep and chronobiology. Curr Neurol Neurosci Rep 2014;14:432.

Reeve K, Bailes B. Insomnia in adults: etiology and management. JNP 2010;6(1):53-60.

Richey SM, Krystal AD. Pharmacological advances in the treatment of insomnia. Curr Pharm Design 2011;17:1471-5.

Rogers RR. Past, present, and future use of oral appliance therapies in sleep-related breathing disorders. J CA Dent Assoc 2012;40(2):151-7.

Roth T, Roehrs T. Sleep organization and regulation. Neurology 2000;54(5) (suppl 1):S2-7.

Ruoff C, Cao M, Guilleminault C. Hypocretin antagonists in insomnia treatment and beyond. Curr Pharm Design 2011;17:1476-82.

Sahar S, Sassone-Corsi P. Metabolism and cancer: the circadian clock connection. Nature 2009;9:886-96.

Sangal RB, Thomas L, Mitler MM. Maintenance of wakefulness test and multiple sleep latency test. Measurement of different abilities in patients with sleep disorders. Chest 1992;101(4):898-902.

Scammel TE, Winrow CJ. Orexin receptors: pharmacology and therapeutic opportunities. Annu Rev Pharmacol Toxicol 2011;51:243-66.

Schutte-Rodin S, Broch L, Buysse D, et al. Clinical guideline for the evaluation and management of chronic insomnia in adults. J Clin Sleep Med 2008;4(5):487-504.

Sehgal A, Mignot E. Genetics of sleep and sleep disorders. Cell 2011;146(2):194-207.

Severino G, Manchia M, Contu P, et al. Association study in a Sardinian sample between bipolar disorder and the nuclear receptor REV-ERBalpha gene, a critical component of the circadian clock system. Bipolar Disord 2009;11(2):215-20.

Soria V, Martinez-Amorós E, Escaramis G, et al. Differential association of circadian genes with mood disorders: CRY1 and NPAS2 are associated with unipolar major depression and CLOCK and VIP with bipolar disorder 2010;35(6):1279-89.

Stahl SM. Stahl's essential psychopharmacology: neuroscientific basis and practical applications. 4th ed. New York, NY: Cambridge University Press; 2013.

Stippig A, Hübers U, Emerich M. Apps in sleep medicine. Sleep Breathing 2015;19(1):411-7.

Tafti M. Genetic aspects of normal and disturbed sleep. Sleep Med 2009;10:S17-21.

Tafti M, Dauvilliers Y, Overeem S. Narcolepsy and familial advanced sleep-phase syndrome: molecular genetics of sleep disorders. Curr Opinion Genetics Dev 2007;17:222-7.

Tahara Y, Shibata S. Chrono-biology, chrono-pharmacology, and chrono-nutrition. J Pharmacological Sci 2014;124:320-35.

Takahashi S, Hong HK, McDearmon EL. The genetic of mammalian circadian order and disorder: implications for physiology and disease. Nat Rev Genetics 2008;9(10):764-75.

Takao T, Tachikawa H, Kawanishi Y, et al. CLOCK gene T3111C polymorphism is associated with Japanese schizophrenics: a preliminary study. Eur Neuropsychopharmacol 2007;17(4):273-6.

Tarasiuk A, Reuveni H. The economic impact of obstructive sleep apnea. Curr Opinion Pulmonary Med 2013;19(6):639-44.

Thaiss CA, Zeevi D, Levy M, et al. Transkingdom control of microbiota diurnal oscillations promotes metabolic homeostasis. Cell 2014;159:514-29.

Thorpe AJ, Clair A, Hochman S, et al. Possible sites of therapeutic action in restless legs syndrome: focus on dopamine and α2δ ligands. Eur Neurol 2011;66:18-29.

Thorpy MJ, Dauvilliers Y. Clinical and practical consideration in the pharmacologic management of narcolepsy. Sleep Med 2015;16(1):9-18.

Trotti LM, Saini P, Bliwise DL, et al. Clarithromycin in gamma-aminobutyric acid-related hypersomnolence: a randomized, crossover trial. Ann Neurol 2015;78(3):454-65.

Trotti LM, Saini P, Freeman AA, et al. Improvement in daytime sleepiness with clarithromycin in patients with GABA-related hypersomnia: clinical experience. J Psychopharmacol 2013;28(7):697-702.

Van Someren EJ, Riemersma-Van Der Lek RF. Live to the rhythm, slave to the rhythm. Sleep Med Rev 2007;11(6):465-84.

Vgontzas AN, Fernadez-Mendoza J, Bixler EO, et al. Persistent insomnia: the role of objective short sleep duration. Sleep 2012;35(1):61-8.

Wulff K, Gatti S, Wettstein JG, Foster RG. Sleep and circadian rhythm disruption in psychiatric and neurodegenerative disease. Nat Rev Neurosci 2010;11(8):589-99.

Yeoh JW, Campbell EJ, James MH, et al. Orexin antagonists for neuropsychiatric disease: progress and potential pitfalls. Frontiers Neurosci 2014;8(36):1-12.

Zaharna M, Dimitriu A, Guilleminault C. Expert opinion on pharmacotherapy of narcolepsy. Expert Opinion Pharmacother 2010;11(10):1633-45.

Zawilska JB, Skene DJ, Arendt J. Physiology and pharmacology of melatonin in relation to biological rhythms. Pharmacological Rep 2009;61(3):383-410.

Stahl's Illustrated | Index

Optional CME Posttest and Certificate

Release/Expiration Dates
Released: July, 2016
CME Credit Expires: July, 2019

Study Guide

This optional posttest with CME credits is available for a fee, (waived for NEI Members). **NOTE: Posttests can only be submitted online.** The posttest questions have been provided below solely as a study tool to prepare for your online submission. **_Faxed/ mailed copies of the posttest cannot be processed_** and will be returned to the sender. If you do not have access to a computer, contact customer service at 888-535-5600.

1. Regina is a 24-year-old who sleeps approximately 5 hours per night. Her twin sister, Rachel, sleeps approximately 10 hours per night. Which of the following has been associated with an increased risk of diabetes, depression, and death?

   A. Short sleep duration (<7 hours/night)

   B. Long sleep duration (>9 hours/night)

   C. Both of the above

   D. Neither of the above

2. Paul is a 21-year-old college student who is interested in using over-the-counter melatonin to help with his sleep/wake cycle while studying for final exams. Which of the following statements is true regarding endogenous melatonin?

   A. Melatonin is released from the pineal gland during periods of darkness

   B. Melatonin is released from the pineal gland during periods of light

   C. Melatonin is released from the suprachiasmatic nucleus during periods of darkness

   D. Melatonin is released from the suprachiasmatic nucleus during periods of light

3. Steven is a 42-year-old blind individual with retinoblastoma who suffers from non-24 sleep disorder. In healthy, sighted individuals, the majority of light input is received by:

   A. The core region of the suprachiasmatic nucleus

   B. The shell region of the suprachiasmatic nucleus

   C. Hypothalamic nuclei outside of the suprachiasmatic nucleus

4. A 31-year-old patient with narcolepsy with cataplexy demonstrates profound loss of hypocretin/orexin (Hcrt/Ox) neurons in the lateral hypothalamus. Hcrt/Os typically stimulates:

A. Acetylcholine release from the basal forebrain

B. Acetylcholine release from the pedunculopontine nucleus

C. Acetylcholine release from the laterodorsal tegmental area

D. All of the above

E. None of the above

5. Michelle is an obese 37-year-old woman who works the night shift as a toll collector. Recent evidence indicates that a disrupted sleep/wake cycle may increase one's risk for obesity, diabetes, and cardiovascular disease by:

A. Increasing levels of leptin

B. Increasing levels of ghrelin

C. Increasing levels of both leptin and ghrelin

D. Decreasing levels of both leptin and ghrelin

6. A 61-year-old man suffers from advanced sleep phase disorder (ASPD). Polymorphisms in which of the following components of the molecular clock have been associated with ASPD?

A. Circadian locomotor output cycles kaput (CLOCK)

B. Cryptochrome (CRY)

C. Period (PER)

D. Retinoic acid-related orphan receptor (ROR)

7. Anthony is a 52-year-old man who recently underwent diagnostic testing for obstructive sleep apnea. Results show that this patient has an apnea-hypopnea index (AHI) of 17. An AHI of 17 is indicative of:

A. No sleep apnea

B. Mild sleep apnea

C. Moderate sleep apnea

D. Severe sleep apnea

8. A 12-year-old male patient has been brought to the clinic by his parents for evaluation. The patient typically sleeps for 10 or more hours a day (yet still exhibits excessive daytime sleepiness), eats excessive amounts of food, and demonstrates disinhibited behaviors including masturbation in public places. This patient most likely has:

A. Idiopathic hypersomnia

B. Narcolepsy without cataplexy

C. Kleine-Levin syndrome

9. Maureen is a 42-year-old woman with complaints of insomnia. Among the FDA-approved treatments for insomnia are:

A. The benzodiazepine temazepam

B. The antidepressant doxepin

C. The nonbenzodiazepine hypnotic zaleplon

D. The melatonin receptor agonist ramelteon

E. All of the above

10. A 29-year-old male patient with shift work disorder exhibits excessive daytime sleepiness that is interfering with his ability to perform duties as an emergency medical responder. He is initiated on armodafinil with good therapeutic response. Modafinil, and its R-enantiomer armodafinil, are hypothesized to promote wakefulness and increase alertness by:

A. Decreasing norepinephrine

B. Decreasing hypocretin/orexin

C. Increasing histamine

D. All of the above

E. None of the above

11. I commit to making the following change(s) in my practice as a result of participating in this activity.

A. Evaluate sleep/wake disturbances in my patients presenting with mood disorders

B. Evaluate mood disorders in my patients presenting with sleep/wake disorders

C. A and B

D. I am already doing both of the above

Instructions for Optional Posttest and CME Certificate
There is a fee for the optional posttest (waived for NEI Members).

1. Read the book, evaluating the content presented

2. Complete the posttest and evaluation, available only online at **www.neiglobal.com/CME** (under "Book")

3. Print your certificate (if a score of 70% or more is achieved)

Questions? call 888-535-5600, or email CustomerService@neiglobal.com